Salivary Gland Infections

Guest Editors

MICHAEL D. TURNER, DDS, MD, FACS
ROBERT GLICKMAN, DMD

ORAL AND MAXILLOFACIAL SURGERY CLINICS OF NORTH AMERICA

www.oralmaxsurgery.theclinics.com

Consulting Editor
RICHARD H. HAUG, DDS

August 2009 • Volume 21 • Number 3

SAUNDERS an imprint of ELSEVIER, Inc.

W.B. SAUNDERS COMPANY
A Division of Elsevier Inc.

1600 John F. Kennedy Blvd. • Suite 1800 • Philadelphia, PA 19103-2899

www.oralmaxsurgery.theclinics.com

ORAL AND MAXILLOFACIAL SURGERY CLINICS OF NORTH AMERICA Volume 21, Number 3
August 2009 ISSN 1042-3699, ISBN-13: 978-1-4377-1250-6, ISBN-10: 1-4377-1250-9

Editor: John Vassallo; j.vassallo@elsevier.com
Developmental Editor: Theresa Collier

Oral and Maxillofacial Surgery Clinics of North America (ISSN 1042-3699) is published quarterly by Elsevier Inc., 360 Park Avenue South, New York, NY 10010-1710. Months of issue are February, May, August, and November. Business and Editorial Offices: 1600 John F. Kennedy Blvd., Suite 1800, Philadelphia, PA 19103-2899. Periodicals postage paid at New York, NY and additional mailing offices. Subscription prices are $271.00 per year for US individuals, $401.00 per year for US institutions, $125.00 per year for US students and residents, $313.00 per year for Canadian individuals, $478.00 per year for Canadian institutions, $362.00 per year for international individuals, $478.00 per year for international institutions and $170.00 per year for Canadian and foreign students/residents. To receive student/resident rate, orders must be accompanied by name or affiliated institution, date of term, and the *signature* of program/residency coordinator on institution letterhead. Orders will be billed at individual rate until proof of status is received. Foreign air speed delivery is included in all *Clinics* subscription prices. All prices are subject to change without notice. **POSTMASTER:** Send address changes to *Oral and Maxillofacial Surgery Clinics of North America,* Elsevier Periodicals Customer Service, 11830 Westline Industrial Drive, St. Louis, MO 63146. Tel: 1-800-654-2452 (U.S. and Canada); 314-453-7041 (outside U.S. and Canada). Fax: 314-523-5170. E-mail: journalscustomerservice-usa@elsevier.com (for print support); journalsonlinesupport-usa@elsevier.com (for online support).

Reprints. For copies of 100 or more, of articles in this publication, please contact the Commercial Reprints Department, Elsevier Inc., 360 Park Avenue South, New York, NY 10010-1710. Tel.: 212-633-3812; Fax: 212-462-1935; Email: reprints@elsevier.com.

Oral and Maxillofacial Surgery Clinics of North America is covered in MEDLINE/PubMed (*Index Medicus*).

Printed and bound by CPI Group (UK) Ltd, Croydon, CR0 4YY

Transferred to Digital Print 2011

Contributors

CONSULTING EDITOR

RICHARD H. HAUG, DDS
Carolinas Center for Oral Health
Charlotte, North Carolina

GUEST EDITORS

MICHAEL D. TURNER, DDS, MD, FACS
Department of Oral and Maxillofacial Surgery,
New York University College of Dentistry,
New York, New York

ROBERT GLICKMAN, DMD
Department of Oral and Maxillofacial Surgery,
New York University College of Dentistry,
New York, New York

AUTHORS

SHAHID R. AZIZ, DMD, MD
Associate Professor, Department of Oral
and Maxillofacial Surgery, University of
Medicine and Dentistry of New Jersey,
New Jersey Dental School, Newark,
New Jersey

ITZHAK BROOK, MD, MSc
Professor of Pediatrics and Medicine,
Georgetown University School of Medicine,
Washington, DC

ERIC R. CARLSON, DMD, MD, FACS
Professor and Chairman, Department
of Oral and Maxillofacial Surgery; and
Director, Oral and Maxillofacial Surgery
Residency Program, University of Tennessee
Graduate School of Medicine, University of
Tennessee Cancer Institute, Knoxville,
Tennessee

**LUKE CASCARINI, BDS, MBBCh, FDSRCS,
FRCS**
Tonbridge Dental Practice, Tonbridge, Kent;
and Specialist Registrar in Oral and
Maxillofacial Surgery, Queen Victoria Hospital,
East Grinstead, United Kingdom

ROBERT GLICKMAN, DMD
Department of Oral and Maxillofacial Surgery,
New York University College of Dentistry,
New York

GABRIEL HERSHMAN, DDS
Resident, Department of Oral and Maxillofacial
Surgery, New York University-Bellevue
Hospital Center, New York, New York

AMY K. HSU, MD
Department of Otorhinolaryngology, Head
and Neck Surgery, New York Presbyterian
Hospital, Weill Medical College of Cornell
University, New York, New York

HEINRICH IRO, MD
Professor, Chair, and Director, Department
of Otorhinolaryngology, Head and Neck
Surgery, University of Erlangen Nuremberg,
Erlangen, Germany

VASILIKI KARLIS, DMD, MD, FACS
Associate Professor and Director, Advanced
Education Program in OMS, New York
University College of Dentistry, NYU Medical
Center, New York, New York

NILS KLINTWORTH, MD
Resident, Department of Otorhinolaryngology,
Head and Neck Surgery, University of Erlangen
Nuremberg, Erlangen, Germany

DAVID I. KUTLER, MD
The Anne Belcher, MD, Assistant Professor,
Department of Otorhinolaryngology, Head and
Neck Surgery, New York Presbyterian
Hospital, Weill Medical College of Cornell
University, New York, New York

MICHAEL LELL, PhD, MD
Senior Physician, Department of Radiology,
University of Erlangen Nuremberg, Erlangen,
Germany

MARK McGURK, MD, FDSRCS, FRCS, DLO
Head, Department of Oral & Maxillofacial Surgery,
Guy's Hospital, London, United Kingdom

ASHISH PATEL, DDS
Resident in Oral and Maxillofacial Surgery,
Department of Oral and Maxillofacial Surgery,
New York University College of Dentistry, NYU
Medical Center, New York, New York

ANDREA SCHREIBER, DMD
Clinical Professor, Department of Oral and
Maxillofacial Surgery, New York University
College of Dentistry, New York, New York

RABIE M. SHANTI, DMD
Resident, Department of Oral and Maxillofacial
Surgery, University of Medicine and Dentistry
of New Jersey, New Jersey Dental School,
Newark, New Jersey

MICHAEL D. TURNER, DDS, MD, FACS
Department of Oral and Maxillofacial Surgery,
New York University College of Dentistry,
New York, New York

JOHANNES ZENK, MD
Professor and Vice Chairman,
Department of Otorhinolaryngology,
Head and Neck Surgery,
University of Erlangen Nuremberg,
Erlangen, Germany

Contents

> The parotid gland is the salivary gland most commonly affected by inflammation. However, infection of the salivary glands can occur in any of the glands. The most common pathogens associated with acute bacterial infection are *Staphylococcus aureus* and anaerobic bacteria. The predominant anaerobes include: anaerobic Gram negative bacilli (eg, pigmented *Prevotella* and *Porphyromonas*); *Fusobacterium* spp; and *Peptostreptococcus* spp. In addition, *Streptococcus* spp (including *Streptococcus pneumoniae)* and aerobic and facultative Gram-negative bacilli (including *Escherichia coli)* have been reported. Aerobic and facultative Gram-negative bacilli are often seen in hospitalized patients. Organisms less frequently found are *Haemophilus influenzae, Treponema pallidum, Bartonella henselae*, and *Eikenella corrodens. Mycobacterium tuberculosis* and atypical mycobacteria are rare causes of infection. The choice of antibiotics should be guided by identification of the etiologic agent.

> This article presents a survey of the imaging procedures in inflammatory changes of the salivary glands. State-of-the-art procedures are described along with a perspective on recent innovations. Various imaging procedures are discussed, including ultrasound, computed tomography, and magnetic resonance imaging. Then, imaging options in different forms of acute and chronic sialadenitis are considered. The choice of method is guided by consideration of the reliability, the side effects, the accessibility, and, ultimately, the costs. The focus is mainly on diagnostic ultrasound and resonance methods because, with their aid, the investigation of almost all the inflammatory diseases of the large salivary glands can be performed with accurate results, without exposing the patient to radiation.

> Salivary gland infections are frequently encountered entities that are acquired in community and hospital settings. These infections have many causes and may be treated with a diverse array of modalities ranging from conservative medical therapy to removal of the affected salivary gland. Minimally invasive techniques employing diagnostic and interventional sialoendoscopy exist between these two extremes. If possible, the goal of management of such infections is to preserve the gland. It is the purpose of this article to review the diagnosis and treatment of acute and chronic salivary gland infections.

> This article reviews major salivary gland anatomy and the differential diagnosis of salivary gland disease. The surgical technique for parotid and submandibular gland

excision is described in detail. Possible complications and their management are also discussed, followed by a brief literature review of new surgical techniques.

Michael D. Turner

Obstructive disease and chronic infections often are managed by extirpative gland surgery. With the advent of new technology and better understanding of salivary physiology, minimally invasive surgical techniques provide the opportunity for safer and less invasive surgery in alternative care settings and the prospect for gland sparing and restoration of normal function. This article describes techniques for managing acute and chronic salivary gland infections using sialoendoscopy.

Andrea Schreiber and Gabriel Hershman

Historically, the most significant non-HIV viral infection of salivary glands has been, and remains, mumps. Despite the widespread administration of mumps vaccines worldwide, sporadic outbreaks continue to be reported. Epidemiologic studies are invaluable in understanding the etiology of these outbreaks. Information gleaned from these studies, coupled with advances in immunology, virology, and DNA/RNA testing will hopefully result in the development of vaccination regimens to ensure eradication of the disease.

Rabie M. Shanti and Shahid R. Aziz

The authors review the clinical presentation, diagnostic evaluation, and treatment modalities for salivary gland enlargement in an HIV-infected population. Because this can occasionally be the presenting clinical symptom of HIV infection, it is important for the oral/maxillofacial surgeon to diagnose and manage HIV salivary gland enlargement.

Ashish Patel and Vasiliki Karlis

The incidence of salivary gland infections in the pediatric population is low but not infrequently seen in pediatric oral and maxillofacial surgery practices and hospital environs. With an ever increasing armamentarium of diagnostic tools and medical and surgical therapies, these patients can be managed successfully with minimum morbidity and decreased incidence of recurrences.

Luke Cascarini and Mark McGurk

This article approaches sialadenitis from a personal perspective based on 15 years of clinical practice limited mainly to salivary gland diseases. Disorders of the salivary glands are uncommon. When they occur, experience in managing the process is diluted over a range of disciplines. The result is that traditional views go unchallenged and are recast unchanged from one textbook to another. Sialadenitis of bacterial origin is a relatively uncommon occurrence today and is normally associated with sialoliths. The most common viral infection of the salivary glands is mumps.

Michael D. Turner and Robert Glickman

Salivary gland infections arise from a wide variety of etiologies: bacteria, localized viruses, systemic viruses, autoimmune diseases, secondary to sialoliths and strictures, and congenital disorders. When dealing with these entities, the diagnosis of the majority of them can be made quickly, although some of the rarer diseases are more difficult to recognize, particularly when they have a more obvious secondary bacterial infection. This article presents six cases and describes their management.

Oral and Maxillofacial Surgery Clinics of North America

THE CLINICS ARE NOW AVAILABLE ONLINE!

Access your subscription at:
www.theclinics.com

Preface

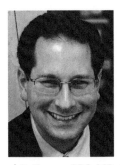
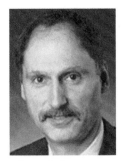

Michael D. Turner, DDS, MD, FACS   Robert Glickman, DMD
Guest Editors

It is our privilege to be the Guest Editors of this issue on the clinical features and etiology of the varying types of salivary infections, and the appropriate management strategies from a historical and present day perspective.

Salivary gland infections are found in at least 1% of the global population, and can be caused by bacterial, viral, and other sources. Salivary gland infections generally have similar features on presentation, although further investigation often reveals the distinct features that distinguish each type and offer clues as to their management. Some are acute in nature and need only palliative or pharmacologic care, while often the pathology is of a long-standing disease requiring more complex and, when appropriate, surgical intervention utilizing the latest technology and rehabilitation to regain function. It is our goal that this issue will become a valued resource that will allow practitioners to review, and if necessary, use as a reference when encountering salivary gland infection pathology.

The organization of this issue begins with bacterial infections, specifically the microbiology. The middle section focuses on viral infections, epidemiology, and pediatric salivary gland infections. The final article is a review of the different diseases in case-presentation format, and provides reinforcement of the principles iterated in each article.

Michael D. Turner, DDS, MD, FACS
Department of Oral and Maxillofacial Surgery
New York University College of Dentistry
345 E. 24th Street
New York, NY 10010

Robert Glickman, DMD
Department of Oral and Maxillofacial Surgery
New York University College of Dentistry
345 E. 24th Street
New York, NY 10010

E-mail addresses:
mdt4@nyu.edu (M.D. Turner)
rsg1@nyu.edu (R. Glickman)

Oral Maxillofacial Surg Clin N Am 21 (2009) ix
doi:10.1016/j.coms.2009.06.001
1042-3699/09/$ – see front matter © 2009 Elsevier Inc. All rights reserved.

The Bacteriology of Salivary Gland Infections

Itzhak Brook, MD, MSc

KEYWORDS

- Sialadenitis • Parotitis • Abscess • Anaerobes
- *Staphylococcus aureus* • Beta-lactamase

Salivary gland infection (SGI) is an acute infection of the salivary glands that can occur in any of the glands and can present as an acute single episode or as multiple recurrent episodes. Sialadenitis is a general term that includes acute, chronic, or recurrent infection and/or inflammation condition affecting the salivary glands. Sialadenitis encompasses a number of conditions that include acute, recurrent, and chronic viral, bacterial, fungal, parasitic and protozoal infections, as well as immunologically mediated diseases, and granulomatous diseases (Giant cell and mycobacterial). The parotid gland is the most frequently involved in SGI; most reports of the microbiology of SGI are devoted to this condition.[1] The microbiology of infection of the submandibular and sublingual glands has rarely been reported.[2]

This review describes the bacterial causes of SGI. Identification of the bacterial etiology of the infection can serve as a guide for the proper selection of antimicrobial therapy for the management of the infection.

PATHOGENESIS
Bacterial Salivary Gland Infections

There are several mechanisms that lead to bacterial SGI.[1] The mode of spread of organisms into the salivary gland may be caused by combinations of factors that enhance ascension of oral bacteria through the salivary ducts, including Stensen's and Wharton's ducts.[2,3] Retrograde contamination of the salivary ducts and parenchymal tissues by bacteria that reside in the oral cavity account for one mechanism. The second mechanism is the stasis of salivary flow through the ducts and parenchyma, which enhances acute or recurrent suppurative infection. Stasis can be caused by hypersalivation, dehydration, medication induced salivary flow reduction, obstruction caused by malignancy, strictures, adhesions and sialolithiasis. Acute suppurative SGI may arise from a septic focus in the mouth, such as chronic tonsillitis or dental sepsis. Another possible mode of transmission of organisms is through transitory bacteremia, especially in the neoatal period. Although these processes can occur in any of the major or minor salivary glands, they most often affect the parotid and submandibular glands.

SGI occurs mostly in newborns[4] and the elderly[5] who are debilitated by systemic illness or previous surgical procedures, although persons of all ages may be affected.

MICROBIOLOGY
Newborns

Speigel and colleagues[6] described two cases of neonatal suppurative parotitis and summarized other 32 patients described in the English literature during the past 35 years. The most common pathogen was *Staphlycoccus aureus*, which was found in 18 (55%) patients. Less common isolates were other Gram-positive cocci (eg, viridans streptococci, *Streptococcus pyogenes, Peptostreptococcus* spp and coagulase-negative *Staphylococcus* spp) (22%); Gram-negative bacilli (*Klebsiella pneumoniae, Escherichia coli*, and *Moraxella catarrhalis*) (16%); and rarely anaerobic bacteria. Aerobic Gram-positive cocci and Gram-negative bacilli were recovered from 94% of the infected glands (**Table 1**).

Georgetown University School of Medicine, 4431 Albemarle Street NW, Washington, DC 20016, USA
E-mail address: ib6@georgetown.edu

Oral Maxillofacial Surg Clin N Am 21 (2009) 269–274
doi:10.1016/j.coms.2009.05.001
1042-3699/09/$ – see front matter © 2009 Elsevier Inc. All rights reserved.

Table 1
Bacterial and mycobacterial pathogens associated with suppurative salivary gland

Organism	Common	Rare

Bacteria	Aerobic bacteria:
	   Staphylococcus aureus
	   Streptococcus pyogenes
	   Alpha-hemolytic streptococci
	Aerobic bacteria:
	   Peptostreptococcus spp
	   Prevotella spp
	   Porphyromonas spp
	   Fusobacterium nucleatum
		Aerobic bacteria:
		   Streptococcus pneumoniae
		   Alpha hemolytic streptococci
		   Haemophilus influenzae
		   Moraxella catarrhalis
		   Pseudomonas aeruginosa
		   Pseudomonas pseudomallei
		   Escherichia coli
		   Proteus spp
		   Salmonella spp
		   Klebsiella spp
		   Actinobacillus spp
		Anaerobic bacteria:
		   Actinomyces spp

Mycobacteria	Mycobacterium tuberculosis Mycobacterium avium-intracellulare Other mycobacteria	—

McAdams and colleagues[7] described a case of a premature neonate who developed suppurative submandibular sialadenitis from a hypervirulent strain of methicillin-resistant *S. aureus* (MRSA). This neonate's hospital-acquired MRSA harbored the Panton–Valentine leukocidin gene (PVL) a well-known virulence factor associated with skin and soft tissue infections, as well as more serious infections. The genes *lukS-PV* and *lukF-PV* (*pvl*) encode the subunits of the Panton–Valentine leukocidin (PVL). MRSA isolates associated with disease bear *pvl* with nearly universal prevalence. The authors also summarized additional 16 cases of neonatal suppurative sialadentitis. Culture of the purulent material grew *S. aureus* in every case (16/17) except one, which grew *Pseudomonas aeruginosa*. Three of the *S. aureus* isolated were MRSA. An additional case of neonatal suppurative sialadentitis caused by non-MRSA was later described by Weibel and colleagues.[8]

Brook[9] described the recovery of anaerobic bacteria from aspirates of an infected salivary gland in two newborns with suppurative sialadenitis and two infants with suppurative parotitis.[10] *Peptostreptococcus intermedius* and *Prevotella melaninogenica* were isolated from one child with left submandibular gland, and *Prevotella intermedia* from the other patient who had a left submandibular gland.[9] In the two cases with paotitis, *Peptostreptococcus magnus, P. intermedia* and *S. pyogenes* were isolated from one newborn and *Prevotella melaninogenica* and *Fusobacterium nucleatum* from the other.[10]

Older Children and Adults

S. aureus is the most common pathogen associated with acute bacterial parotitis and has been cultured in 50% to 90% of cases in older children and adults.[11–14] Of concern was the reported recovery of MRSA from two cases of parotid abscesses.[15] Other causative organisms include streptococci (including *Streptococcus pneumoniae and S. pyogenes*), and *H. influenzae.*[11–14] Gram-negative bacilli (including *E. coli, K. pneumoniae, Salmonella* spp, and *Pseudomonas aeruginosa*) have also been rarely reported.[16,17] In Southeast Asia, *Pseudomonas pseudomallei*, an organism found in soil and surface water, is a frequent cause of acute parotitis, especially in children.[18] Gram-negative organisms are often seen in hospitalized patients.

Organisms less frequently found are: *Mycobacterium tuberculosis* and atypical mycobacteria,[19–26] *Treponema pallidum, Bartonella henselae* (cat-scratch bacillus),[25] and *Eikenella corrodens*.

Cervicofacial actinomycosis is a granulomatous disease mostly caused by *Actinomyces israelii*, which is a strict anaerobe. Less commonly, infection is caused by *Actinomyces propionica, Actinomyces naeslundii, Actinomyces viscosus, Actinomyces eriksonii* and *Actinomyces odontolyticus,* which are all members of the oral bacterial flora. Depending on the composition of the concomitant synergistic flora, the onset of actinomycosis may be acute, subacute, or chronic.[27] When *S. aureus* or beta-hemolytic streptococci are involved, an acute painful abscess or a phlegmatous cellulitis may be the initial manifestation. The salivary glands may be involved by direct extension of an odontogenic source.

Several reports describe anaerobic isolates from parotid infections.[26,28–35] However, the true incidence of anaerobic bacteria in suppurative parotitis has not yet determined because most past studies did not employ proper techniques for their isolation.

Brook and Finegold[32] reported two patients with acute suppurative parotitis In one case, the cultures yielded mixed culture of *P. intermedia* and alpha-hemolytic streptococci. In the other child, no aerobes were recovered and the specimen yielded growth of *F. nucleatum* and *P. intermedius*. Of interest is that both of these patients were institutionalized, mentally retarded children, and one had Down's syndrome. Notably, children with Down's syndrome have a striking incidence of severe periodontal disease and have a greater prevalence of *P. melaninogenica* in the gingival sulcus in comparison with normal children.[36]

Sussman[33] recovered *Gaffkya anaerobia* from recurrently infected parotid gland. *A. israelii* and *A. eriksonii* also have been isolated.[31]

Brook and colleagues[17] studied 23 aspirates of pus from acute suppurative parotitis for aerobic and anaerobic bacteria. A total of 36 bacterial isolates (20 anaerobic and 16 aerobic and facultative) were recovered, accounting for 1.6 isolates per specimen (0.9 anaerobic and 0.7 aerobic and facultative). Anaerobic bacteria only were present in 10 (43%) patients, aerobic and facultatives in 10 (43%), and mixed aerobic and anaerobic flora in 3 (13%). Single bacterial isolates were recovered in nine infections, six of which were *S. aureus* and three of which were anaerobic bacteria. The predominant bacterial isolates were *S. aureus* (eight isolates), anaerobic Gram-negative bacilli (six isolates, including four pigmented *Prevotella* and *Porphyromonas*), and *Peptostreptococcus* spp (five).

Aspirates of pus from acute suppurative sialadenitis were studied for aerobic and anaerobic bacteria (**Table 2**).[10] Bacterial growth was present in a total of 47 specimens: 32 from parotid, nine from submandibular, and six from sublingual glands specimens. A total of 55 isolates (25 aerobic and 30 anaerobic) were recovered from parotid infection; anaerobic bacteria only were recovered in 13 (41%); aerobic or facultative bacteria only in 11 (34%); and mixed aerobic and anaerobic bacteria were recovered in 8 (25%). A total of

Table 2
Bacterial isolates in 47 acute suppurative sialadenitis

Bacteria Isolated	Parotid Gland (n = 32)	Submandibular Gland (n = 9)	Sublingular Gland (n = 6)
Aerobic and facultative bacteria			
Streptococcus pneumoniae	3	1	—
Streptococcus pyogenes	2	1	—
Staphylococcus aureus	10	4	3
Haemophilus influenzae	4	1	—
Escherichia coli	2	—	1
Alpha hem. streptococcus	4	1	1
Subtotal	25	8	5
Anaerobic bacteria			
Peptostreptococcus spp	9	3	3
Actinomyces israelii	2	1	—
Proprionbacterium acnes	4	1	—
Eubacterium lentum	2	—	1
Fusobacterium spp	4	1	—
Bacteroides spp	2	—	—
Prevotella spp	5	2	1
Porphyromonas assacharolytica	2	1	—
Subtotal	30	9	5
Total	55	17	10

From Brook I. Aerobic and anaerobic microbiology of suppurative sialadenitis. J Med Microbiol 2002;5:526; with permission.

17 isolates (eight aerobic and nine anaerobic) were recovered from submandibular gland infection; anaerobic bacteria only were recovered in three (33%) specimens; aerobic or facultative bacteria only in four (44%); and mixed aerobic and anaerobic bacteria were recovered in two (22%). A total of 10 isolates (five aerobic and five anaerobic) were recovered from sublingual gland infection; anaerobic bacteria only were recovered in two (33%) specimens; aerobic or facultative bacteria only in two (33%); and mixed aerobic and anaerobic bacteria were recovered in two (33%). The predominant aerobic bacteria were *S. aureus* and *H. influenzae* and the predominate anaerobes were Gram negative bacilli (including pigmented *Prevotella* and *Porphyromonas*, and *Fusobacterium* spp) and *Peptostreptococcus* spp. This study highlights the polymicrobial nature and importance of anaerobic bacteria in acute suppurative sialadenitis.

There are two other reports of recovery of anaerobes from infections of other salivary glands. Bock[37] described a patient with sublingual gland inflammation and a bad taste in the mouth. Numerous spirochetes and a few fusiform bacilli were seen on smears. Baba and colleagues[38] obtained an anaerobic Gram-positive coccus in pure culture from a purulent submandibular gland infection.

THE PATHOGENESIS OF SALIVARY GLAND INFECTION DUE TO ANAEROBIC BACTERIA

Although acute SGI caused by anaerobic bacteria has been infrequently reported, its occurrence should not be surprising. Both clinicopathologic correlations in humans and experimental studies in dogs have shown that bacteria can ascend Stensen's duct from the oral cavity and thus infect the parotid gland.[39] Improved techniques for isolation and identification of anaerobic bacteria have shown that the flora of the mouth is predominantly anaerobic, and normal adults harbor about 10^{11} microorganisms per gram of material in gingival crevices.[40] Saliva contains many genera of anaerobic bacteria, including *Peptostreptococcus, Veillonella, Actinomyces, Propionibacterium, Leptotrichia*, pigmented *Prevotella* and *Porphyromonas, Bacteroides*, and *Fusobacterium* spp. Diminution in salivary flow could allow the ascent of any of the indigenous bacterial flora, thereby triggering acute parotitis.[34]

Pigmented *Prevotella* and *Porphyromonas* spp are the most common anaerobic Gram-negative bacilli found in oral flora and, like *Peptostreptococcus* spp, they are frequently isolated from odontogenic and orofacial infections.[41] These

infections include tonsillar, peritonsillar, and retropharyngeal abscesses, cervical lymphadenitis, chronic sinusitis, and intracranial infections.[42] The paucity of reports of involvement of these organisms in bacterial SGI is probably because anaerobic cultures were not performed, or because of the lack of adequate anaerobic transport or culture techniques.

IDENTIFICATION OF ORGANISMS

Expression of the pus from the parotid gland and performance of Gram stain may support suppurative infection. Specimens for anaerobic culture should not be taken from the Stensen's duct because oropharyngeal contamination is certain. Cultures of blood can also reveal the causative organisms. However, the abscess or infected site may harbor more organisms then those isolated from the blood.

Needle aspiration of the purulent gland may yield the causative organism. If no pus is aspirated, introduction of sterile saline and subsequent aspiration may yield organisms. The aspirates should be cultured and special stains should be performed for aerobic as well as anaerobic bacteria, fungi, and mycobacteria.

Isolation of anaerobic organisms is optimized by transporting the aspirated pus in a syringe or a special transport media supportive of anaerobic bacteria.[43] These are preferred to use of a swab. Pus specimens transported to the laboratory in a syringe should be plated on medium supportive of anaerobic growth within 20 minutes of collection. Surgical exploration and drainage may be indicated for diagnosis as well as for therapy.

The most valuable investigation for *Mycobacterium* spp is a fine needle aspiration biopsy, which frequently can confirm the suspected diagnosis, and avoid the sequelae of excisional surgery, such as fistula formation. Histologic examination of the biopsied material can confirm the diagnosis. Polymerase chain reaction (PCR) testing of aspirate can assist in identifying mycobacterium[44] as well as *B. henselae*.[45]

SUMMARY

The most common pathogens associated with acute SGI are *S.aureus* and anaerobic bacteria. The predominant anaerobes include Gram-negative bacilli (ie, *Prevotella* and *Porphyromonas* spp), *Fusobacterium* spp, and *Peptostreptococcus* spp. Additionally, *Streptococcus* spp (including *S. pneumoniae* and *S.pyogenes*) and aerobic and facultative Gram-negative bacilli (including *E. coli*) have been reported. Aerobic and facultative Gram-negative organisms are often seen in hospitalized patients. Organisms less frequently found are: *H. influenzae, K. pneumoniae, Salmonella* spp, *P. aeruginosa, T. pallidum, B. henselae.,* and *E. corrodens.* Mycobacterium tuberculosis and atypical mycobacteria are rare causes of parotitis. Adequate identification of the microorganisms that cause SGI allows for proper of selection of antimicrobial therapy.

REFERENCES

1. Krippaehne WW, Hunt TK, Dunphy JE. Acute suppurative parotitis: a study of 161 cases. Ann Surg 1962; 156:251–7.

2. Petersdorf RG, Forsyth BR, Bernanke D. *Staphylococcal parotitis.* N Engl J Med 1958;259:1250–8.

3. Seifert G. Aetiology and histological classification of sialadenitis. Pathologica 1997;89:7–17.

4. Pershall KE, Koopmann CF, Coulthard SW. Sialadenitis in children. Int J Pediatr Otorhinolaryngol 1986;11:199–203.

5. Pajukoski H, Meurman JH, Odont D, et al. Salivary flow and composition in elderly patients referred to an acute geriatric ward. Oral Surg Oral Med Oral Pathol Oral Radiol Endod 1997;84:265–71.

6. Spiegel R, Miron D, Sakran W, et al. Acute neonatal suppurative parotitis: case reports and review. Pediatr Infect Dis J 2004;23:76–8.

7. McAdams RM, Mair EA, Rajnik M. Neonatal suppurative submandibular sialadenitis: case report and literature review. Int J Pediatr Otorhinolaryngol 2005;69:993–7.

8. Weibel L, Goetschel P, Meier R, et al. Neonatal suppurative submandibular sialadenitis. Neonatal suppurative submandibular sialadenitis. Pediatr Infect Dis J 2005;4:378–80.

9. Brook I. Suppurative sialadenitis associated with anaerobic bacteria in newborns. Pediatr Infect Dis J 2006;25:280.

10. Brook I. Aerobic and anaerobic microbiology of suppurative sialadenitis. J Med Microbiol 2002;51: 526–9.

11. Saarinen RT, Kolho KL, Pitkäranta A. Cases presenting as parotid abscesses in children. Int J Pediatr Otorhinolaryngol 2007;71:897–901.

12. Brook I. Diagnosis and management of parotitis. Arch Otolaryngol Head Neck Surg 1992;118: 469–71.

13. Feinstein V, Musher DM, Young EJ. Acute bilateral suppurative parotitis due to *Haemophilus influenzae;* report of two cases. Arch Intern Med 1979; 139:712–3.

14. Rousseau P. Acute suppurative parotitis. J Am Geriatr Soc 1990;38:897–8.

15. Mohammed I, Hofstetter M. Acute bacterial parotitis due to methicillin-resistant *Staphylococcus aureus.* South Med J 2004;97:1139.

16. Masters RG, Cormier R, Saginur R. Nosocomial gram-negative parotitis. Can J Surg 1986;29:441–2.

17. Brook I, Frazier EH, Thompson DH. Aerobic and anaerobic microbiology of acute suppurative parotitis. Laryngoscope 1991;101:170–2.

18. Dance DA, Davis TM, Wattanagoon Y, et al. Acute suppurative parotitis caused by *Psuedomonas pseudomallei* in children. J Infect Dis 1989;159:654–60.

19. Bhat NA, Stansbie JM. Tuberculous parotitis: a case report. J Laryngol Otol 1996;110:976–7.

20. O'Connell JE, Speculand GB, Pahor AL. Mycobacterial infection of the parotid gland: an unusual cause of parotid swelling. J Laryngol Otol 1993;107:561–4.

21. Perlman DC, D'Amico R, Salomon N. Mycobacterial infections of the head and neck. Curr Infect Dis Rep 2001;3:233–41.

22. Holmes S, Gleeson MJ, Cawson RA. Mycobacterial disease of the parotid gland. Oral Surg Oral Med Oral Pathol Oral Radiol Endod 2000;90:292–8.

23. Handa U, Kumar S, et al. Tuberculous parotitis: a series of five cases diagnosed on FNAC. J Laryngol Otol 2001;115:235–7.

24. Hira SK, Hira RS. Parotitis with secondary syphilis. Br J Vener Dis 1984;60:121–2.

25. Malatskey S, Fradis M, Ben-Davis J, et al. Cat-Scratch disease of the parotid gland. Ann Otol Rhinol Laryngol 2000;109:679–82.

26. Anthes WH, Blaser MJ, Reller B. Acute suppurative parotitis associated with anaerobic bacteremia. Am J Clin Pathol 1981;75:260–2.

27. Oostman O, Smego RA. Cervicofacial actinomycosis: diagnosis and management. Curr Infect Dis Rep 2005;7:170–4.

28. Shevky M, Kohn C, Marshall MS. *Bacterium melaninogenicum.* J Lab Clin Med 1934;19:689.

29. Heck WE, McNaught RC. Periauricular infection, probably arising in the parotid. JAMA 1952;149: 662–3.

30. Beigelman PM, Rantz LA. Clinical significance of *Bacteroides.* Arch Intern Med 1949;84:605.

31. Hensher R, Bowerman J. Actinomycosis of the parotid gland. Br J Oral Maxillofac Surg 1985;23: 128–34.

32. Brook I, Finegold SM. Acute suppurative parotitis caused by anaerobic bacteria: report of two cases. Pediatrics 1978;62:1019.

33. Sussman SJ. *Gaffkya anaerobia* infection and recurrent parotitis. Clin Pediatr 1986;25:323–4.

34. Lewis MA, Lamey PJ, Gibson J. Quantitative bacteriology of a case of acute parotitis. Oral Surg Oral Med Oral Pathol 1989;68:571–5.

35. Guardia SN, Cameron R, Phillips A. Fatal necrotizing mediastinitis secondary to acute suppurative parotitis. J Otolaryngol 1991;20:54–6.

36. Meskin LH, Farsht EM, Anderson DL. Prevalence of *Bacteroides melaninogenicus* in the gingival crevice area of institutionalized trisomy 21 and cerebral palsy patients and normal children. J Periodontol 1968;39:326–8.

37. Bock E. Ueber isolierte Entzundung der Glandula sublingualis durch Plaut-Vincentsche Infektion. Munch Med Wochenschr 1938;85:786–8 [German].

38. Baba S, Mamiya K, Suzuki A. Anaerobic bacteria isolated from otolaryngologic infections. Jpn J Clin Pathol 1971;19(Suppl):35–8.

39. Berndt AL, Buck R, Buxton RL. The pathogenesis of acute suppurative parotitis. Am J Med Sci 1931;182:639–40.

40. Socransky SS, Manganiello SD. The oral microbiota of man from birth to senility. J Periodontol 1971;42:485–6.

41. Finegold SM. Anaerobic bacteria in human disease. New York: Academic Press; 1977.

42. Brook I. Anaerobic bacteria in upper respiratory tract and other head and neck infections. Ann Otol Rhinol Laryngol 2002;111:430–40.

43. Jousimies-Somer HR, Summanen P, Baron EJ, et al. Wadsworth-KTL anaerobic bacteriology manual. 6th edition. Belmont (CA): Star Publishing; 2002.

44. Kim YH, Jeong WJ, Jung KY, et al. Diagnosis of major salivary gland tuberculosis: experience of eight cases and review of the literature. Acta Otolaryngol 2005;125:1318–22.

45. Ridder GJ, Richter B, Laszig R, et al. Parotid involvement in cat scratch disease: a differential diagnosis with increased significance. Laryngorhinootologie 2000;79:471–7.

Diagnostic Imaging in Sialadenitis

Johannes Zenk, MD[a],*, Heinrich Iro, MD[a], Nils Klintworth, MD[a],
Michael Lell, PhD, MD[b]

KEYWORDS

- Sialadenitis • Imaging • CT • MRI Ultrasound
- Salivary glands

Inflammation of the large salivary glands in humans is, usually, relatively easy to recognize clinically because of the symptoms, swelling, and pain. On one hand, the history, palpation, and inspection certainly enable a coarse differentiation to be made regarding the localization and cause of the disease. On the other hand, imaging procedures lead to swifter verification of the diagnosis and to adequate therapeutic results, which are thus obtained more quickly.

In the diagnosis and treatment of salivary gland inflammation, apart from otolaryngologist and oral and maxillofacial surgeons, pediatricians and general physicians are also involved. In many countries, diagnostic imaging generally consists of conventional sialography, CT, and MRI. In central Europe, diagnostic ultrasound and color Doppler ultrasound are part of the training curriculum of otolaryngologist and oral and maxillofacial surgeons. Thus in many centers, ultrasound examination of the large salivary glands is also in prominent use. The survey of the imaging procedures in inflammatory changes of the salivary glands that is presented here is intended to describe the state-of-the-art procedures and to provide a perspective on recent innovations. This article, therefore, is focused mainly on the emphasis on diagnostic ultrasound and resonance methods because, with their aid, the investigation of almost all the inflammatory diseases of the large salivary glands can be performed with accurate results, without exposing the patient to radiation. The diagnostic gap that remains with the two procedures is filled by the modern procedure of sialoendoscopy. (See the article elsewhere in this issue on sialoendoscopy.)

In the department at Erlangen, approximately 1000 patients attend annually with unclear swellings of the salivary glands, over half of them with an inflammatory, mostly obstructive, cause of the basic symptomatology.

IMAGING PROCEDURES
Conventional Radiology

The use of plain radiographs in the diagnosis of inflammatory diseases of the salivary glands and in the diagnosis of salivary calculi in particular, largely, has faded. Eighty percent to 95% of calculi in the submandibular gland are radio-opaque[1,2] and 60% to 70% of calculi in the parotid gland can only be demonstrated by using high-resolution radiograph films (**Fig. 1**).[3,4] In the differential diagnosis, adhesions, strictures and vascular malformations must be considered, in addition to sialoliths (**Fig. 2**).[5] Calcified lymph nodes, scars, and arteriosclerotic changes may be seen on the radiographs and may be mistaken for salivary calculi.

Conventional Sialography

Since it was first performed by Arcelin[6] in 1921, conventional sialography has been the established procedure of choice for demonstrating the excretory ducts of the large salivary glands and the technique has changed little to date. The sialographic equipment includes a water-soluble,

a Department of Otorhinolaryngology, Head and Neck Surgery, University of Erlangen Nuremberg, Waldstrasse 1, D-91054 Erlangen, Germany
b Department of Radiology, University of Erlangen Nuremberg, Maximiliansplatz 1, D-91054 Erlangen, Germany
* Corresponding author.
E-mail address: johannes.zenk@uk-erlangen.de (J. Zenk).

Oral Maxillofacial Surg Clin N Am 21 (2009) 275–292
doi:10.1016/j.coms.2009.04.005

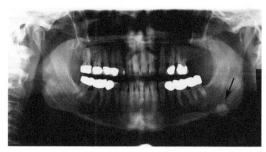

Fig. 1. Sialolith (*arrow*) of a l/r submandibular gland in native radiograph.

nonionic contrast agent, a set of dilators (0.016 in for Wharton's duct, 0.035 in for Stensen's duct), a sialographic cannula, a polyethylene connecting tube, and a 5 mL syringe. Once the orifice is identified, the cannula should be gently advanced into the orifice to avoid perforation. Then the contrast agent is slowly injected using manual pressure. After injecting 1.5 to 4.0 mL of contrast agent, radiographs are obtained. Ten minutes after removing the cannula, delayed phase images may be obtained.

Typical signs of chronic recurrent sialadenitis are an irregularly enlarged (sausage-shaped) main duct and pruning of the distal ducts; calculi may be present. In Sjögren's syndrome (myoepithelial sialadenitis), nonobstructive sialectasia can be found. However, because of its invasiveness, the method does have risks (injuries to the excretory duct system, possible allergic reactions, and acute infections of the gland).[7] Acute sialadenitis is considered a contraindication to sialography. Noninvasive procedures such as diagnostic ultrasound[8,9] and MRI with magnetic resonance (MR)-sialography[10,11] are pushing conventional sialography increasingly into the background. CT sialography is allocated only a secondary role in

view of its invasiveness and the exposure to radiation.[12,13]

In our own department, conventional sialography was no longer employed for routine investigation in over 500 patients with obstructive sialadenitis. Nevertheless, in one of the few publications in the last 5 years, Ngu and colleagues[14] regard sialography as being particularly important in the evaluation of stenoses of the ducts (**Fig. 3**).

Ultrasound

The salivary glands can be excellently demonstrated with modern high-resolution ultrasound equipment because of their superficial location. Even so, the quality of the ultrasound examination depends on the operator. However, by integrating diagnostic ultrasound and color Doppler ultrasound into the training plans for otolaryngologist and oral and maxillofacial surgeons a high level of competence can be ensured. An exact knowledge of the clinical picture facilitates the diagnostic classification of the findings by the practiced ultrasound operator. Inflammatory changes in the glands are described as the ideal indication for diagnostic ultrasound.[15]

The simplest type of examination is performed with the patient supine and the head slightly hyperextended. The hyperextension is particularly important in the examination of the submandibular gland, so that the ultrasound transducer for the examination of the hilar region of the gland can be placed parallel to the horizontal lower jaw: this is the exact method by which abnormalities of the excretory duct can be identified (70% of submandibular calculi are situated in this

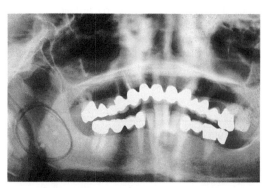

Fig. 2. Radiograph of an arteriovenous malformation within the right caudal parotid gland: calcified lesions (*circle*) no sialoliths.

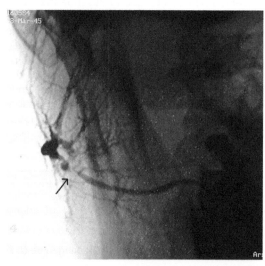

Fig. 3. Stenosis of Stensen's duct (*arrow*) in sialography.

region).[15–18] To render the classification of the pathologic findings more comprehensible, the normal findings of the parotid, submandibular, and sublingual glands are described.

The parotid appears as a smooth bordered, homogeneous, echo-rich organ. The anterior regions of the gland and the accessory glands are related to the masseter muscle and can be differentiated from the more hypoechoic buccal fatty tissue by the contraction and relaxation of the chewing musculature. The dorsal boundary is formed by the mastoid and the sternocleidomastoid muscle and, caudally, the posterior belly of the digastric muscle. The retromandibular vein can be demonstrated in the gland parenchyma, (**Fig. 4**). Intraparotid lymph nodes are only detectable if enlarged.

The submandibular gland extends cranially to the lower jaw and the mylohyoid muscle. It surrounds these in an arch and frequently extends anteromedially as far as the sublingual gland. It is crossed laterally by the facial vein and artery, easily demonstrable by ultrasound. The ultrasound image of the submandibular gland, like that of the other glands, is homogeneous and echo-rich. There are no lymph nodes situated within the gland parenchyma (**Fig. 5**).

The sublingual gland lies beneath the mucosa of the floor of the mouth, near the lingual frenulum. The gland is bordered anteriorly and medially by the geniohyoid and genioglossus muscles, and caudally by the mandible. The short excretory duct is not normally demonstrable (**Fig. 6**).

Demonstrating Stensen's duct and Wharton's duct is generally only performed for obstructions and disorders of salivary flow (**Figs. 7** and **8**). However, demonstrating the ducts plays a considerable role in the investigation of inflammatory salivary gland diseases because obstructive sialadenitis is the most frequent form of

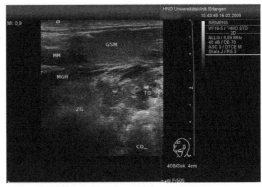

Fig. 5. Submandibular gland, normal finding in ultrasound. CO, oral cavity; GSM, submandibular gland; MGH, geniohyoid muscle; MM, mylohyoid muscle; TO, tonsillar region; ZG; root of tongue.

inflammation. A few important suggestions that can facilitate exploration of the duct system are:

Knowledge of the anatomy.
High-frequency ultrasound transducers with tissue harmonic imaging (THI)-mode (**Fig. 9**A, B).
No excessive pressure by the transducer because, particularly in Stensen's duct, this leads to compression of the lumen of the excretory duct and renders it invisible.
In the case of Wharton's duct, the position of the transducer should be parallel to the horizontal part of the mandible.
The administration of oral vitamin C as a sialagogue can markedly improve visualization of the duct after 20 seconds even in cases of only relative duct obstruction (**Fig. 10**A, B).[19]

The image acquisition has a very significant influence on the later interpretation of the results. The following parameters are essential in ensuring the objectification of the findings:[18]

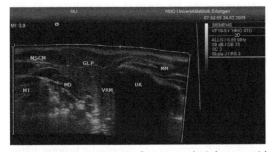

Fig. 4. Panorama image of a normal right parotid gland. GLP, parotid gland; MD, posterior belly of digastric muscle; MM, masseter muscle; MSCM, sternocleidomastoid muscle; MT, trapezoid muscle; UK, mandible; VRM, retromandibular vein.

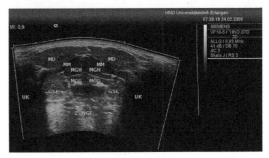

Fig. 6. Normal sublingual gland. GSL, sublingual gland; MD, anterior belly of digastric muscle; MGG, genioglossal muscle; MGH, geniohyoid muscle; MM, mylohyoid muscle; UK, mandible; ZUNGE, tongue.

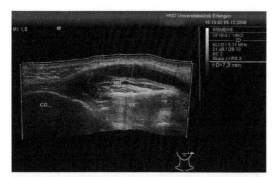

Fig. 7. Dilated left mega-Stenseńs duct (+...+) caused by a scarred stenosis. CO, oral cavity; MM, masseter muscle; UK, mandible.

Guiding the transducer must be accurately defined. In a transverse examination, the left side of the monitor image corresponds to the right side of the patient and, in a longitudinal examination, the left side on the monitor corresponds to the structures lying cranially.

At the beginning of every ultrasound examination, image adjustment of the equipment should be performed for the individual patient.

The examination should be performed in a standard sequence and the recording of the images should include anatomic landmarks to aid orientation. A pictogram for the transducer position and later image interpretation is indispensable.

In paired organs such as the large salivary glands, it is important to compare the lateral symmetry of the echo structure.

Since the beginning of diagnostic ultrasound in the head and neck region in the 1980s, the technical equipment has developed much farther and

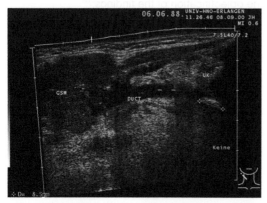

Fig. 8. Dilated Whartońs duct over the whole floor of the mouth visible as an echo-free band, caused by a distally located sialolith (+...+). GSM, submandibular gland; UK, mandible.

the image quality, the classification of the findings, and the ability to objectify have improved markedly. It is beyond doubt that, in principle, a valid investigation of the salivary glands can beperformed with a 7.5 MHz transducer and a B-scan (brightness) machine. To optimize the informative value, the following technical details must be available:

Ultrasound device with two scanners with variable frequencies (7.5 MHz–10.0 MHz, and 11 MHz–14 MHz) to record both deep and superficial structures with a high resolution. The higher the frequency, the better the resolution, but the poorer the depth of penetration. Thus, localized masses above a diameter of 3 mm are demonstrable. Because of the large leap in impedance, calculi can already be detected by ultrasound above a size of 1.5 mm to 2 mm (**Fig. 11**).[20]

Color Doppler function to recognize the vasculature and circulatory pattern in the gland (Question: excretory duct or vessel—increased blood flow in Sjögren's disease) (**Fig. 12**).[21]

Panorama imaging: wider section images than in CT, hence better classification of findings (see **Fig. 4**).

Using the harmonics of the reflected sound, such as in THI, to improve the resolution (see **Fig. 9**A, B).

CT and CT Sialography

Nonenhanced CT is the most sensitive imaging modality for detecting calculi within the duct system or the glandular parenchyma. The inferior soft-tissue resolution of CT makes it difficult to visualize the nondilated duct system. To overcome this problem, the technique of CT sialography, a combination of conventional radiograph sialography and CT scanning, has been introduced and proposed by several investigators in the preoperative evaluation of salivary gland tumors.[22–24] Three-dimensional images of the duct system can be rendered, but the spatial resolution is inferior to conventional radiograph or digital subtraction sialography, and the procedure exposes the patient to additional radiation. The advent of high-resolution MR sialography has widely replaced this technique. Intravenous contrast material administration is indicated to visualize inflammatory or neoplastic lesions within the salivary glands, and to detect areas of abscess formation.

Nonenhanced CT or CT sialography can be performed with the following parameters: 120 kV, 80

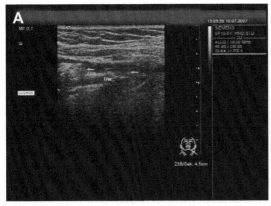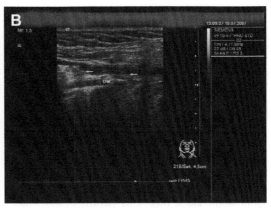

Fig.9. (*A*) Unclear swelling of a left submandibular gland with combined dilation of the duct. DW, Whartoń's duct. (*B*) THI allows a better resolution of the structures: mylohyoid muscle (*arrows*).

to 100 mAs, slice thickness less than 1 mm; image reconstruction with high resolution algorithm at 0.3 to 0.5 mm intervals; individually adapted field of view (< 200 mm); and scan range determined by the glandular anatomy. Contrast-enhanced CT can be performed at 120 kV, 160 to 200 mAs, slice thickness < 1 mm, 3 mm thick images reconstructed with a soft tissue algorithm at 3 mm intervals, individually adapted field of view (< 200 mm), thin slice images may be reconstructed for three-dimensional reformations. The scan range should cover the gland and the thoracic inlet in patients with a suspicion of abscess formation to rule out mediastinal involvement.

MRI and MR-sialography

MRI is the preferred imaging modality after ultrasound for evaluating salivary gland lesions, though may not be indicated for the evaluation of sialoliths, particularly if they are nonobstructive. Saliva has a very high-signal intensity on T2-weighted (T2w) images and acts like an endogenous contrast material. Without cannulation of the main duct and injection of contrast material, Wharton's and Stensen's duct can be visualized with heavily T2w sequences: single-shot turbo spin echo (TSE), rapid acquisition with relaxation enhancement (RARE), half-Fourier acquisition single-shot TSE (HASTE), and single-slab 3D TSE sequence with slab-selective, variable excitation pulse (SPACE). High-field MR systems (1.5–3.0 Tesla) systems with dedicated surface coils provide excellent spatial resolution. A typical examination consists of axial T1-weighted (T1w) images before and after IV injection of a gadolinium-based contrast material, T2w images with fat saturation, coronal T1w images with fat saturation, and one of the above-mentioned MR sialography sequences. Diffusion-weighted imaging may be performed additionally. The slice thickness of the conventional MR sequences (except MR

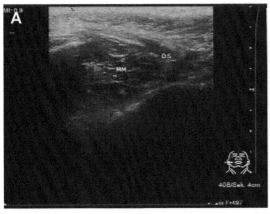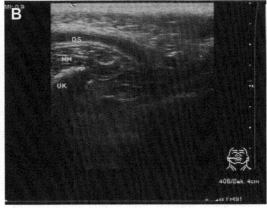

Fig.10. Dilation of a right Stensen's duct (+...+) caused by a stenosis before (*A*) and after (*B*) stimulation of saliva with vitamin C. DS, Stenseń's duct; MM, masseter muscle; UK, mandible.

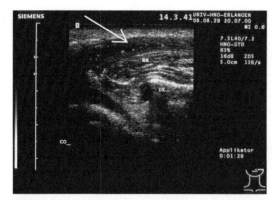

Fig. 11. Single stone fragments (*arrow*) below 1-mm diameter after lithotripsy of a stone within the left Stensenś duct. CO, oral cavity; MM, masseter muscle; UK, mandible.

sialography) should not exceed 3 to 5 mm. Functional information on the gland can be obtained by oral application of lemon juice,[25] 5% citric acid[10] or tartaric acid[26] in patients with xerostomia.

Scintigraphy

Scintigraphy involves the afferent and efferent flow of radioactive 99m pertechnetate that, besides the thyroid gland and the tear ducts, is mainly taken up by the salivary glands following IV administration. Here Tc-99m is transferred into and out of the cells by transport mechanisms in place of chloride ions. By this means, quantitative data on the function of the salivary glands can be obtained relating to the kinetics of this uptake and release. In addition, visual comparison of the uptake between the thyroid and the salivary glands provides a qualitative, subjective assessment.[27] One problem with

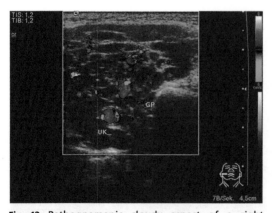

Fig. 12. Pathognomonic cloudy aspect of a right parotid gland together with intense blood flow in color-coded sonography. GP, parotid gland; UK, mandible.

scintigraphy is the quantification and comparability of the findings. Currently this is still the objective of detailed research projects.[28] Hence salivary gland scintigraphy tends, as a rule, to be employed in measuring the function of the gland during studies[29–31] or during treatment. A lower enrichment in the gland parenchyma can be anticipated in radiation sialadenitis and in Sjögren's disease with xerostomia, whereas in obstructive sialadenitis there is persistent activity in the parenchyma on the affected side (**Fig. 13**). The method has less relevance in clinical routine.

IMAGING IN DIFFERENT DISEASES

The indication for imaging is dependent on the symptomatology and clinical picture of the patient. In each case, it will be preceded by a clinical examination of the salivary glands, including palpation (also bimanual) and massage of the glands to detect calculi, if present, or to assume, based on the composition of the saliva, an inflammation or an obstruction in the case of the absence of saliva. The choice of method is guided by consideration of the reliability, the side effects, the accessibility, and, ultimately, the costs. As already mentioned, the large salivary glands are exceptionally suitable for ultrasound imaging in view of their easy accessibility and their superficial location. As this is directly and rapidly available, at reasonable cost and without side effects, in the authors' opinion this is the method of choice in diagnostic investigation. In our own department, over 95% of cases of sialadenitis could be clarified definitively by this means and treated appropriately. Diagnostic ultrasound can also be used reliably in children and can be repeated during and after therapeutic interventions. If a reliable diagnosis is not achieved by ultrasound, then MRI or MR sialography is indicated as a further noninvasive procedure. CT should only be used in individual cases, such as unclear findings on ultrasound or contraindications for MRI. If necessary, the investigations can be augmented by sialoendoscopy (see the article by Turner elsewhere in this issue). Disease pictures with their clinical characteristics and the findings are discussed in detail below.

Acute Viral and Bacterial Sialadenitis and Salivary Gland Abscess

Acute viral sialadenitis can be caused by the mumps virus, cytomegalovirus, or less common viruses. Often a bilateral painful swelling of the glands is detectable clinically. The typical ultrasound finding is an echo-homogeneous gland swelling (**Fig. 14**) and, in cases involving the

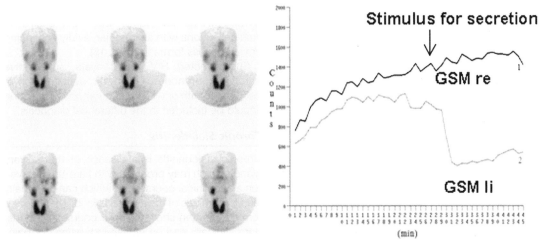

Fig. 13. Szintigramm and time-intensity curves of the salivary glands. Note the missing decrease of intensity after stimulation within the right submandibular gland (GSM re); whereas the left submandibular gland (GSM li) shows loss of intensity after stimulation.

parotid gland, the presence or absence of more hypoechoic areas that correspond to enlarged lymph nodes. In the differential diagnosis, it is necessary to consider sialadenosis or bulimia, which is accompanied by bilateral swelling of the parotid gland.

When isolated echo-poor changes are detected, which correspond to lymph nodes (**Fig. 15**), these are not reliable guides for the differential diagnosis.

In the case of acute bacterial sialadenitis, diagnostic ultrasound in the early stages demonstrates a diffuse enlargement of the entire diseased gland, such as in viral parotitis. Here the organ is well demarcated from the adjacent structures. Later

the parenchymal pattern usually appears looser, inhomogeneous, coarser, and more hypoechoic. These findings are attributable to the edematous swelling of the organ; that is, to the increased fluid content of the inflamed parenchyma. The excretory duct system filled with pus is often well demonstrated in cases of purulent sialadenitis (**Fig. 16**). Areas of softening appear echo-poor to echo-free with an echo-rich rim and with marked dorsal sound reinforcement. Echoes of ill-defined masses in the center of these softening lesions can represent necrotic areas of tissue. If further softening takes place, anechoic areas can occur with partly sharp and partly blurred demarcation, which then represent an abscess (**Fig. 17**). If

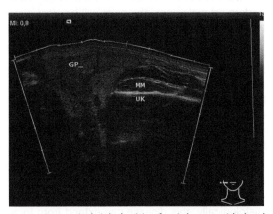

Fig. 14. Acute viral sialadenitis of a right parotid gland with echo-homogenic signal of the parenchyma and echo-poor signals inside the gland that represent edema of the interstitial space (no ducts). GP, parotid gland; MM, masseter muscle; UK, mandible.

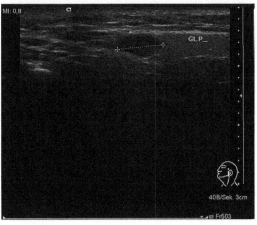

Fig. 15. Reactive lymphadenitis (+…+) at the superior border of the parotid gland (GLP) with a slight echo-rich hilum in its center.

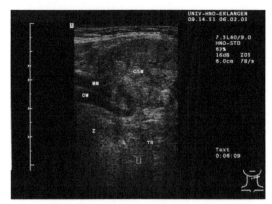

Fig. 16. Acute purulent sialadenitis of a left submandibular gland with dilation of the duct, echo-inhomogenic reflexes, and enlarged gland. DW, Whartoń's duct; GSM, submandibular gland; MM, mylohyoid muscle; TR, tonsillar region; Z, tongue.

necessary, color Doppler examination can distinguish between a highly inflamed, echo-poor area that still has a good blood circulation and an abscess with absent circulation in the center.[15]

CT and MRI are rarely performed in acute (viral) sialadenitis. On CT or MR images, the inflamed gland can be seen as enlarged or of abnormal (hyperdense) attenuation or intensity (high-signal intensity on T2w images), and contrast-enhanced. Contrast enhancement may be more pronounced in bacterial sialadenitis than in viral sialadenitis. Inflammatory stranding of the adjacent soft tissues will usually be present. The presence of enlarged locoregional or intraglandular lymph nodes may suggest inflammation, but can also be seen with neoplasms. One should always search for a sialolith as the underlying cause for sialadenitis; CT is more

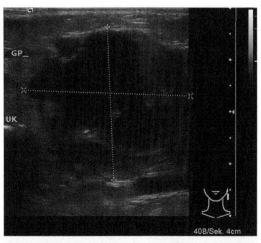

Fig. 17. Abscess formation (+…+) of the left caudal parotid gland with possible origin within a lymph node in a 2-month-old girl. GP, parotid gland; UK, mandible.

sensitive than MRI in demonstrating small calculi. CT and MRI perform equally well in demonstrating fluid collections with an irregular, avidly enhancing rim in abscess formation (**Fig. 18**).

Superinfected HIV-related cysts, suppurative parotid lymph nodes, and cystic degeneration of neoplasms with or without superimposed infection should be included in the differential diagnosis.

Chronic Sialadenitis

Chronic sialadenitis is a disease of the salivary glands which may progress with flare-ups or even run a subclinical course, and which can eventually lead to cirrhosis of the affected gland. The different forms can often show a similar course and signs, both clinically and on ultrasound: painful or painless, recurrent swellings of the affected glands, sometimes with acute exacerbations that then resemble the picture of acute sialadenitis.[32] Nevertheless, typical characteristics of the individual diseases can also be distinguished in the imaging. The appearance of the ultrasonic image is dependent to a large degree on the duration and extent of the inflammation in the gland parenchyma. Usually, there is a marked coarsening in the echotexture and the internal structure appears inhomogeneous, probably because of fibrotic scarring of the parenchyma. Additionally, small cystic areas develop that represent localized duct ectasia. Occasionally, intraglandular microcalcification is visible as echodense structures with dorsal sound shadowing; these should not be mistaken for the typically intraductal sialoliths (**Fig. 19**).

Hallmarks of chronic recurrent sialadenitis are an irregularly enlarged (sausage-shaped) main duct and central ductal dilatation tapering to normal peripheral ducts. If the peripheral ducts and acini are not visualized on a technically well-performed sialogram, the acini will be destroyed and saliva production will decrease, promoting further sialadenitis. The changes in the central duct system may also be appreciated on CT or MR sialography. Diffuse enlargement with or without dystrophic calcifications, associated with low-density areas (pus or dilated intraglandular ducts) are frequent findings. Surrounding fasciitis and lymph node enlargement are usually not present. Fatty infiltration, ductectasia, and volume loss are features of the late stage (**Fig. 20**).

Chronic sclerosing sialadenitis of the submandibular gland, synonym: Küttner tumor

Histologically, this disease can extend from focal sialadenitis to complete cirrhosis of the gland. Typically it occurs in patients between 40 and 70 years of age and mostly affects the submandibular gland, often affecting only one part of the gland.[33]

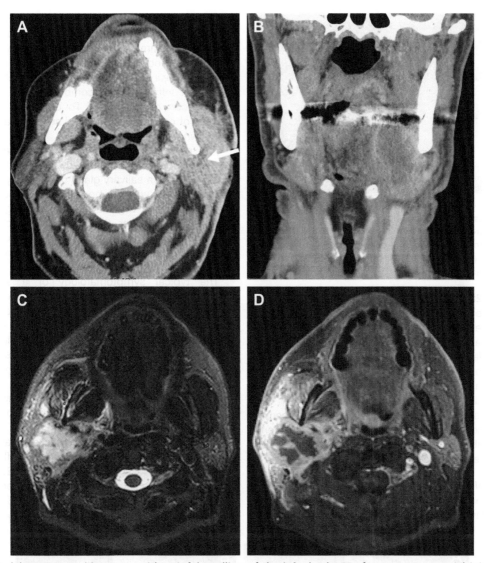

Fig. 18. (*A*) A 72-year-old woman with painful swelling of the left cheek. CT after contrast material injection demonstrates enlarged parotid gland with indistinct borders and diffuse enlargement of the muscles of the masticator space. Low-density area (*arrow*) indicates beginning abscess formation. Note stranding of the subcutaneous fat. *Staphylococcus aureus* was isolated in this patient with acute sialoadenitis. (*B*) A 64-year-old man with abscess formation in the left submandibular gland. (*C*) A 37-year-old man with abscess formation of the right parotid gland. (*D*) T2w image shows fluid collections, the abscess membranes enhance avidly on T1w images with fat saturation after contrast medium injection.

However, even accessory glands of the parotid and the parotid gland itself can be affected (**Fig. 21**). On ultrasound, examination there is a more hypoechoic, rather poorly demarcated mass, which can also affect just parts of the gland parenchyma.[34] In the differential diagnosis the other forms of chronic sialadenitis and particularly tumors of the glands must be considered.

Juvenile recurrent parotitis
This type of inflammation, of which the detailed cause is still unclear (genetic predisposition, malformation of the excretory ducts, congenital duct ectasia, immunopathological processes, IgA deficits), is subdivided into a juvenile form (ages 2 to 13 years) and an adult form with the peak age between 30 and 40 years. Painful swellings of one or both parotids recur with acute purulent episodes at varying intervals and, in the later clinical course, firm swellings. Diagnostic ultrasound demonstrates the typical image with an inhomogeneous echo pattern and also echo-rich and echo-poor areas that can represent ductal ectasia, congested parenchyma, or also lymph nodes

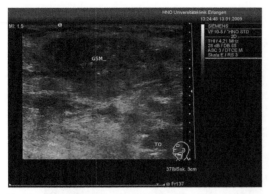

Fig. 19. Chronic obstructive sialadenitis with echo-rich reflexes probably due to microcalcifications within the parenchyma, in a 90-year-old woman with symptoms for years. Note the echo-poor structure of the whole parenchyma. GSM, submandibular gland; TO, tonsillar region.

(Fig. 22A, B).[18,35,36] Very often both glands are affected to a different extent, starting with lymph node enlargement and extending to the complete picture. Diagnostic ultrasound has almost completely displaced sialography, with the pathognomonic finding: "the tree in leaf." CT and MRI demonstrate nonspecific enlargement of the parotid glands, with variable density or SI.[34]

Possible differential diagnoses include Boeck's disease, Sjögren's disease, or a specific sialadenitis. Salivary calculi disease or lymphoma should also be considered.

Chronic obstructive sialadenitis

Obstructive sialadenitis is the most frequent non-neoplastic cause of swellings of the salivary glands. Here, stenosis is mostly caused by a calculus and less often by duct stenoses or webs of inflammatory origin. Occasionally there are foreign bodies or the excretory duct suffers iatrogenic injury, leading to obstructive sialadenitis.[37] Not infrequently a combination of all the factors can be observed. To date, the actual causes of calculi formation and stenoses are still unknown.

The most frequent cause of sialolithiasis is a macroscopically visible calculus formation or calcification in a salivary gland or a salivary gland excretory duct, with the most variable proportions of inorganic and organic matrix. The larger the calculus, the higher the content of inorganic matrix[38] and the more easily it is demonstrable by imaging. Salivary calculi, in principle, can occur in all the large salivary glands in humans.

The typical symptomatology of a salivary calculus colic with postprandial swelling and pains points the examiner in the direction of the diagnosis of sialolithiasis; but asymptomatic calculi occur as an incidental finding in approximately 1% of radiograph examinations by dentists. Over and beyond this, it is important in imaging that complications of acute sialadenitis due to sialolithiasis, such as abscesses, diffuse inflammation of the soft tissues, or sialocutaneous and sialooral fistulae are recognized.

The characteristic direct diagnostic ultrasound criterion for a concretion is an echo-rich reflection with marked dorsal sound shadowing (**Fig. 23**A–C). Although the dorsal sound shadow is regularly demonstrable, occasionally the echo-rich reflection is not clear or is not recognizable. This phenomenon

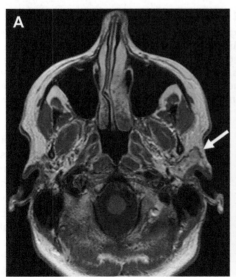

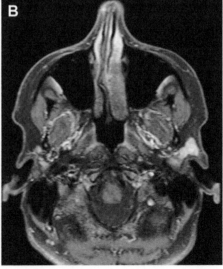

Fig. 20. Focal slightly hyperintense mass (*arrow*), T1w (*A*), in the left parotid gland with homogenous contrast enhancement (*B*), T1w fat saturated + Gadolinium. Histology revealed chronic fibrosing sialoadenitis.

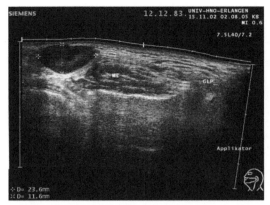

Fig. 21. Chronic sclerotizing sialadenitis (+...+) of an accessory parotid gland within the left cheek of a 22-year-old man. The parotid gland (GLP) shows a hyperechogenic parenchyma as a sign of chronic changes there. MB, masseter muscle.

occurs because the reflected fraction of the ultrasound wave does not reach the transducer or, owing to the surface composition of the calculus, it is dispersed out of the plane of the image; or else the organic part of the calculus does not reflect the ultrasound. Congestion in the excretory ducts can be a further indirect sign of calculus disease, even in the absence of evidence of concretions (see **Figs. 7–9**). Here, duct endoscopy can provide further information as to whether a small calculus or a stenosis is present. Calculi in the large salivary glands are reliably demonstrable by diagnostic ultrasound, owing to the large leap in impedance, from a size of 1.5 mm to 2 mm.[20] From the differential therapeutic point of view, the exact determination of the site of the sialolith (intraglandular, extraglandular, or intraductal) is of great importance. Therefore, it is

essential for the examiner to describe, apart from the size of the calculus, its exact localization within the excretory duct system. The main site for calculi in Wharton's duct, which in 80% of cases is the duct affected, is the hilar region (comma area) in 57%, the distal duct system in 34%, and the gland itself in 9%. Parotid calculi are found in the intraparenchymal duct system in 23% of cases, in the hilus of the gland in 13%, and in the distal Stensen's duct in 64%. It is important for the examiner to note that multiple calculi are found in up to 13% of patients, and bilateral calculi are found in 1%. Salivary calculi can even occur in children under 9 years of age.[17,38]

In the differential diagnosis, consideration must be given to calcified lymph nodes associated with tuberculosis, intraparenchymal microcalcifications, phleboliths, vascular malformations (calcifications), and scarring. Common ultrasound misdiagnoses include the upper horn of the hyoid bone and an elongated styloid, which similarly show up as echo-rich lesions with distal sound shadowing.[18]

Calculi can be easily also detected with nonenhanced CT, which is the most sensitive technique of detecting stones (**Fig. 24**A). Dilatation of the obstructed duct results in a linear hypodense structure abruptly terminated. Swelling of the gland and indistinct morphology are sequels of duct obstruction.

The obstructed duct appears bright and dilated on MR sialography and a "black dot" represents the underlying calculus (see **Fig. 24**B). Swelling of the gland and indistinct definition of the lobules can be seen as described above. Inflammation of the gland produces further swelling and high intensity streaks in the periphery of the gland on T2w

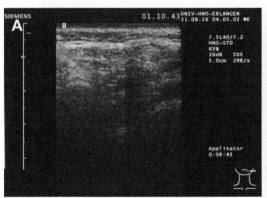

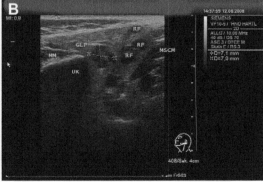

Fig. 22. (*A*) Endpoint of a chronic sialadenitis in an adult of a left parotid gland with no normal parenchymal echo structure: hyper- and hypoechogenic signals in the parotid region. (*B*) Chronic recurrent juvenile parotitis in a 4-year-old boy with recurrent swelling of the both glands. Nodular aspect of the gland, a little echo-poor aspect of the parenchyma with multiple hypoechogenic lesions (RF) with up to 8 mm. GLP, parotid gland; MM, masseter muscle; MSCM, sternocleidomastoid muscle; UK, mandible.

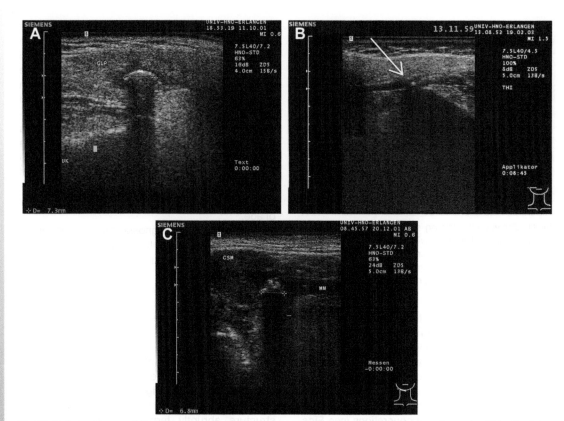

Fig. 23. Salivary stones of the parotid and gland (*A*) echo-rich signal with distal shadow (+…+) within the intra-parenchymatous duct system of a left parotid gland. GLP, parotid gland; UK, mandible. (*B*) 1.5 mm stone of the left parotid. Dilation of Stenseńs duct is better visible than the echo-rich signal of the stone (*arrow*). (*C*) Stone (+…+) within the hilum of a right submandibular gland—a location where most of stones are found. GSM, submandibular gland; MM, mylohyoid muscle.

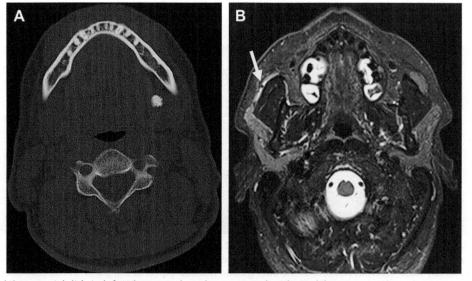

Fig. 24. (*A*) Large sialolith in left Wharton's duct demonstrated with CT. (*B*) Stones are less obvious on MR, but stimulated high resolution MRS can detect even small stones (*arrow*).

images. If the inflammation progresses to abscess formation, fluid collection with a thick surrounding, contrast-enhancing wall can be seen on T2w and T1w images after contrast injection. Stenoses of the main salivary ducts can be accurately detected with MR sialography with a reported sensitivity of 100%, a specificity of 93% to 98%, a positive predictive value of 87% to 95%, and a negative predictive value of 100%. The sensitivity, specificity, and positive and negative predictive values of MR sialography for detecting calculi in this study were 91%, 94% to 97%, 93% to 97%, and 91%, respectively.[39]

Diagnostic ultrasound for intraoperative imaging and postoperative follow-up in obstructive sialadenitis

Of all the advantages of diagnostic ultrasound, the most significant are its immediate availability and its repeatability. Hence, this method is outstandingly suitable for use in certain duct-preserving procedure techniques; for instance, as an intraoperative navigational aid.[40] Moreover, the success of the procedure can be determined immediately postoperatively.[38,41,42]

In extracorporeal shock-wave lithotripsy, diagnostic ultrasound is used for focusing on the calculus and for the post-treatment assessment of the fragmentation (see **Fig. 11**).[42,43] The use of baskets, forceps, and probes for retrieving calculi can be monitored by ultrasound during the intervention (**Fig. 25**). During a difficult incision into a duct, small scissors and forceps can be guided transorally onto the calculus with external ultrasound monitoring, and the success of the procedure can be checked during the intervention (**Fig. 26**A, B). Also, the positioning and direction of advance of the endoscope (eg, in duct stenoses) can be excellently steered by means of intraoperative ultrasound. The subsequent positioning of the stent to keep the stenosis open can be monitored without problems. MRI is sometimes problematic in the early posttraumatic or postsurgical stage if extensive edema in the surrounding soft tissues is present. Lacerations of the ducts, strictures, or fistula formation can be well visualized in the chronic stage (**Fig. 27**).

Other Forms of Chronic Sialadenitis

Pneumoparotitis

Pneumoparotitis is a rare disease and occurs through air insufflation into the excretory duct of the parotid gland (up to 150 mm Hg). As a result, there is a painful recurrent unilateral or bilateral swelling of the parotid gland, which develops within minutes. This is possible, for example, in glassblowers and in brass instrumentalists

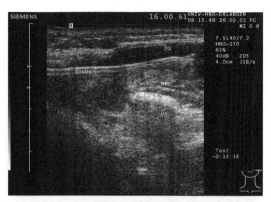

Fig. 25. Probe (*Sonde*) within a dilated Stensen's duct after having passed a stenosis of a left parotid gland, DS, Stensen's duct; MM, masseter muscle; UK, mandible.

(dilatation of Stensen's duct has been demonstrated in sialography). This can also occur in children through strong nose-blowing or blowing up balloons or playing wind instruments.[44]

On ultrasound examination, the air inclusions are detectable as echo-rich reflexes in the duct system with marked sound shadowing and movement on sonopalpation (**Fig. 28**). On CT scanning, the air inclusions are clearly identifiable in the duct, in the gland, and, occasionally, in the surroundings. The CT examination can be performed with a provocation test (blowing out the cheeks) to amplify the effect.

Radiation-induced sialadenitis

Radiation sialadenitis is provoked by irradiation such as in external radiotherapy of head or neck tumors or radioiodine therapy of thyroid gland processes. The first changes are noticeable with a dose of 6Gy.[45] The early reaction causes a painful glandular swelling by damage to the periductal capillary vessels, leading to edema and obstruction of the smaller excretory ducts. On diagnostic ultrasound, the glands appear anechoic at this stage. Through the associated reaction of the surrounding glandular tissue, marked anechoic lines vertical to the skin surface are detectable as signs of lymphoedema. In the CT and MRI, the gland initially appears to be swollen by edema. The take-up of contrast medium is markedly increased in comparison to a normal gland (**Fig. 29**).[46] Functional MR sialography provides an indication of the secreting ability of the gland.[26] If later glandular atrophy occurs, there is echo-inhomogeneity, but most often an echo-richer transformation of the gland parenchyma with a marked reduction in volume.[46]

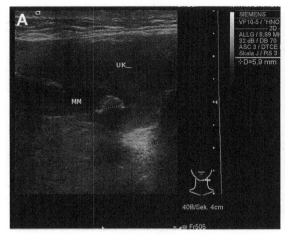
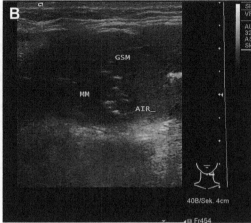

Fig. 26. A 6-mm stone within the hilum of a left submandibular gland before (*A*) and after (*B*) transoral removal. Note the echo-rich reflexes of the air-filled stone region after removal. Altogether dark parenchyma is a sign of obstructive disease. AIR, air reflection; GSM, submandibular gland; MM, mylohyoid muscle; UK, mandible.

Myoepithelial sialadenitis (Sjögren's disease, Sjögren's syndrome)

This autoimmune disease of the salivary glands is referred to as primary Sjögren's syndrome. It mainly affects women, with a peak age of 40 to 50 years. Apart from the sicca symptomatology (dry eyes, mouth, and nose), a salivary gland swelling is detectable in 60% of cases. The involvement of other organ systems is relevant for imaging and clinical care arthritis and other collagenotic symptoms (50%), Raynaud's phenomenon (35%), and, above all, the 44-fold higher risk than the normal population of developing lymphoma (5%–6% B-cell lymphoma,

MALT-lymphoma). In the investigation of Sjögren's disease, sialography and scintigraphy have been regarded as the gold standard up to now.[8] A quantitative standardized assessment using scintigraphic methods can be achieved by calculating the maximum activity and the rate of decrease in activity after stimulation.[47] The conventional sialogram shows nonobstructive sialectasia. Four stages can be differentiated: 1, punctuate contrast collections (< 1 mm); 2, globular contrast collection (1–2 mm); 3, cavitary-contrast collection (> 2 mm); and 4, destruction of the gland parenchyma.[48]

In recent years, diagnostic ultrasound, MRI, or MR sialography have clearly gained in importance. MR demonstrates an inhomogeneous honeycomb-like

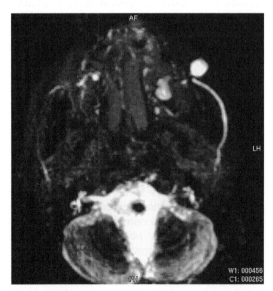

Fig. 27. Sialocele and fistula formation of Stensen's duct after stone extraction.

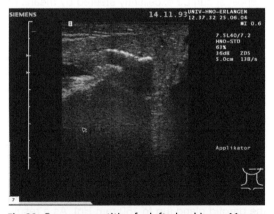

Fig. 28. Pneumoparotitis of a left gland in an 11-year-old boy, who complained of swelling and pain after inflation of a balloon. Hyperechogenic reflexes, which move during investigation, resemble air bubbles in the salivary ducts.

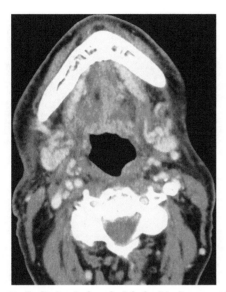

Fig. 29. Radiation-induced sialadenitis in a patient with oropharyngeal carcinoma 1.5 months after completion of radiochemotherapy (with a cumulative dose of 70 Gy). Increased contrast enhancement of the glands and dilated intraglandular ducts within both submandibular glands. Stranding of the subcutaneous fat is caused by lymphatic stasis.

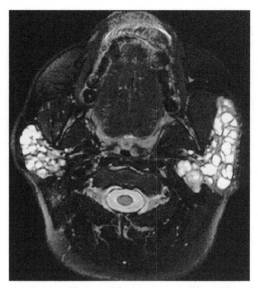

Fig. 30. A 56-year-old woman with Sjögren's syndrome. Multiple cystic lesions >2 mm have replaced most of the glandular parenchyma of both parotid glands. No solid masses are visible.

pattern, sometimes referred to as a "salt and pepper" appearance on T2-weighted and gadolinium-enhanced (Gd)-enhanced T1 weighted images (Fig. 30). Because patients with Sjögren's disease have an elevated risk of salivary gland lymphoma, the glands must be evaluated for the presence of solid masses.

On diagnostic ultrasound, the diseased salivary glands appear enlarged, with an inhomogeneous structure, and echo-poor. There are numerous focal echo-poor masses, which on the one hand can represent cystic dilatation of ducts, but on the other hand may be enlarged intraglandular lymph nodes. Overall, there is a "cloudy" structure (see Fig. 12).

Shimizu and colleagues[9] were able to demonstrate that the ultrasound criteria for diagnostic imaging of Sjögren's disease have exactly the same informational value as sialographic criteria. Multiple echo-poor areas that are surrounded by echo-rich lines and patches or a totally echo-poor gland with blurred demarcation, are suitable criteria for making the diagnosis of Sjögren's disease in the early stage. There is a good correlation with sialography. Nevertheless, it is also emphasized that experienced examiners are clearly better at making the diagnosis. In prospective observations, they achieved a specificity of maximum 94%, a sensitivity of 65%, and a maximum accuracy of 74%. Salaffi and

colleagues[8] arrived at the same result in a large multicenter crossover study: diagnostic ultrasound is more suitable for the diagnosis of Sjögren's disease than sialography and scintigraphy. The authors call for the integration of diagnostic ultrasound into the criteria for the investigation of Sjögren's syndrome of the American European Consensus group.[8]

Boeck's disease (Heerfordt's syndrome, epithelioid cell sialadenitis)

This disease is regarded as a systemic granulomatous inflammation of unclear cause, which seldom only primarily affects the salivary glands—usually the parotid gland. The symptoms of Heerfordt's syndrome include pyrexia, uveitis, and parotitis. The lungs and mediastinal lymph nodes are also frequently affected. The typical symptom as regards the salivary glands is an occasionally painful swelling. On diagnostic ultrasound there is a typical parenchymal pattern with diffuse echo-poor areas spread throughout the gland (Fig. 31), which represent enlarged lymph nodes or affected glandular structures.[49] The image is similar to that of Sjögren's disease or of chronic recurrent juvenile parotitis. Multiple granulomas can be found with sarcoidosis on CT and MR imaging. If the lesion is solitary, the differential diagnosis of a neoplasm always needs to be taken into account. A different presentation is a diffuse enlargement of the gland with homogenous contrast enhancement (Fig. 32).

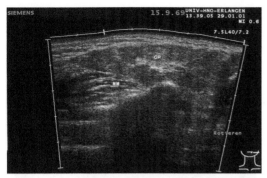

Fig. 31. Sarcoidosis of the parotid glands in a young male adult. Echo-poor and slightly nodulous appearance of the parenchyma together with echo-rich reflexes. It resembles chronic juvenile parotitis or Sjögren's disease. GP, parotid gland; MM, masseter muscle.

Tuberculosis

Tuberculous sialadenitis (pathogen: *Mycobacterium tuberculosis*) with primary or secondary manifestations in the lymph nodes of the parotid gland has certainly become rare nowadays and is more a problem of the developing countries. However, in the last few years, mycobacteria other than tuberculosis (MOTT) are encountered more and more frequently.[50] Particularly in children with symptoms of a hardening of the gland with swelling and occasionally with the development of a fistula, this diagnosis must be taken into account. Apart from the echo-poor enlargement of the gland demonstrated on diagnostic ultrasound, typically enlarged intraparotid lymph nodes are also visible (sometimes massively enlarged). An obstruction in the duct is not usually detectable (**Fig. 33**). Seventy percent of tuberculosis affect the parotid gland, 27% the submandibular gland, and only 3% the sublingual glands.[51] There are two different clinical presentations: one similar to acute sialadenitis, with imaging features similar to acute sialadenitis and abscess formation; the other similar to a salivary gland tumor.

In the differential diagnosis, sialadenitis and lymph node swellings due to other causes such as actinomycosis or lymphoma or metastatic disease must be distinguished.

Enlargement of the salivary glands in bulimia or anorexia, obesity, and sialadenosis

Patients frequently present with bilateral swelling of the parotid and submandibular salivary glands. Usually, it is possible to exclude inflammatory causes, apart from mumps. The pathophysiology of the painless, bilateral swelling of the salivary glands in association with obesity, bulimia, and anorexia has multiple causes. Usually the parotid

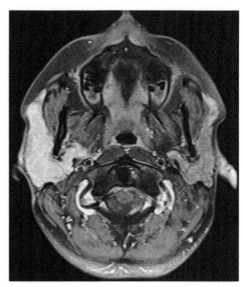

Fig. 32. Sarcoidosis of the right parotid gland—diffuse pattern with enlargement of the gland and homogenous contrast enhancement (T1w fs +Gd).

glands are affected and not the submandibular glands. Obesity and eating disorders clearly differ in respect of the pathogenesis of the parotid swelling. In obese persons, fatty tissue is evidently laid down in the parotid gland tissue; whereas in eating disorders, binge eating and purging, for example, cause demonstrable parenchymal histologic changes. Hormonal influences (T3, T4, GH, ghrelin, leptin) similarly play a role in the disease symptomatology; however, they do not adequately explain the degree and extent of the symptoms. Also, the pathogenesis in so-called

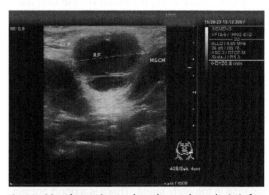

Fig. 33. Mycobacterium other than tuberculosis infection in the left parotid gland of a 2-year-old girl. A 20 mm diameter echo-poor lesion with septa (RF) shows up within the parenchyma of the parotid gland representing an infected and massively enlarged intraparotoid lymph node. GLP, parotid gland; MSCM, sternocleidomastoid muscle.

sialadenosis is frequently attributed to these influences. Diagnostic ultrasound demonstrates a diffuse echo-rich, but homogeneous, enlargement of the glands in all these cases, with no echo-poor zones or lymph node swellings (see **Fig. 27**).[52]

On sialography, the gland is enlarged, and the ducts are of normal caliber, but spread out because of the increase in gland volume. This appearance allows differentiation between chronic sialadenitis and Sjögren's syndrome. CT and MR findings are unspecific and may show increased density (acinar hypertrophy, fibrosis) or decreased density (fatty infiltration) and corresponding signal changes on MR.

REFERENCES

1. Isacsson G, Isberg A, Haverling M, et al. Salivary calculi and chronic sialoadenitis of the submandibular gland: a radiographic and histologic study. Oral Surg Oral Med Oral Pathol 1984;58(5):622–7.
2. Lustmann J, Shteyer A. Salivary calculi: ultrastructural morphology and bacterial etiology. J Dent Res 1981;60(8):1386–95.
3. Perrotta RJ, Williams JR, Selfe RW. Simultaneous bilateral parotid and submandibular gland calculi. Arch Otolaryngol 1978;104(8):469–70.
4. Suleiman SI, Hobsley M. Radiological appearances of parotid duct calculi. Br J Surg 1980;67(12):879–80.
5. Hopkins R. Submandibular sialolithiasis with a case of a cavernous haemangioma presenting as a salivary calculus. Br J Oral Surg 1969;6(3):215–21.
6. Arcelin L. Radiographie d'un calcul salivaire de la glande sublinguale. Lyon Méd 1921;118:769–73 [French].
7. Petridis C, Ries T, Cramer MC, et al. MR-Sialographie: Prospektive Evaluation ultraschneller Sequenzen mit paralleler Bildgebung und oraler Stimulation bei Patienten. RöFo 2007;179(2):153–8 [German].
8. Salaffi F, Carotti M, Iagnocco A, et al. Ultrasonography of salivary glands in primary Sjögren's syndrome: a comparison with contrast sialography and scintigraphy. Rheumatology (Oxford) 2008;47(8):1244–9.
9. Shimizu M, Okamura K, Yoshiura K, et al. Sonographic diagnostic criteria for screening Sjögren's syndrome. Oral Surg Oral Med Oral Pathol Oral Radiol Endod 2006;102(1):85–93.
10. Tanaka T, Ono K, Ansai T, et al. Dynamic magnetic resonance sialography for patients with xerostomia. Oral Surg Oral Med Oral Pathol Oral Radiol Endod 2008;106(1):115–23.
11. Astreinidou E, Roesink JM, Raaijmakers CP, et al. 3D MR sialography as a tool to investigate radiation-induced xerostomia: feasibility study. Int J Radiat Oncol Biol Phys 2007;68(5):1310–9.
12. Szolar DH, Groell R, Preidler K, et al. Three-dimensional processing of ultrafast CT sialography for parotid masses. AJNR Am J Neuroradiol 1995;16(9):1889–93.
13. Jager L, Menauer F, Holzknecht N, et al. Sialolithiasis: MR sialography of the submandibular duct—an alternative to conventional sialography and US? Radiology 2000;216(3):665–71.
14. Ngu RK, Brown JE, Whaites EJ, et al. Salivary duct strictures: nature and incidence in benign salivary obstruction. Dentomaxillofac Radiol 2007;36(2):63–7.
15. Brown J, Greess H, Zenk J, et al. Diagnostic and imaging methods. In: Nahlieli O, editor. Modern management preserving the salivary glands. Herzeliya, Israel: Isradon; 2007. p. 29–67.
16. Iro H. Sonography of the large salivary glands. In: Valvassori GE, Magee MF, Carter BL, editors. Imaging of the head and neck. Stuttgart: Thieme; 1995. p. 500–8.
17. Zenk J, Constantinidis J, Kydles S, et al. Klinische und diagnostische Befunde bei der Sialolithiasis. HNO 1999;47(11):963–9 [German].
18. Iro H, Uttenweiler V, Zenk J. Kopf-Hals-Sonographie. Eine Anleitung zur praxisbezogenen Ultraschalluntersuchung. 1st edition. Berlin: Springer; 2000. p. 167.
19. Bozzato A, Zenk J, Hertel V, et al. Salivary stimulation with ascorbic acid enhances sonographic diagnosis of obstructive sialadenitis. J Clin Ultrasound 2009;37(6):329–32.
20. Födra C, Kaarmann H, Iro H. Sonographie und Röntgennativaufnahme in der Speichelsteindiagnostik - experimentelle Untersuchungen. HNO 1992;40(7):259–65 [German].
21. Shimizu M, Okamura K, Yoshiura K, et al. Sonographic diagnosis of Sjögren syndrome: evaluation of parotid gland vascularity as a diagnostic tool. Oral Surg Oral Med Oral Pathol Oral Radiol Endod 2008;106(4):587–94.
22. Mancuso A, Rice D, Hanafee W. Computed tomography of the parotid gland during contrast sialography. Radiology 1979;132(1):211–3.
23. Som PM, Biller HF. The combined CT-sialogram. Radiology 1980;135(2):387–90.
24. Kassel EE. CT sialography, Part I: Introduction, technique, anatomy, and variants. J Otolaryngol Suppl 1982;12:1–10.
25. Habermann CR, Graessner J, Cramer MC, et al. MR-Sialographie: Optimierung und Bewertung ultraschneller Sequenzen mit paralleler Bildgebung und oraler Stimulation. RöFo 2005;177(4):543–9 [German].
26. Wada A, Uchida N, Yokokawa M, et al. Radiation-induced xerostomia: objective evaluation of salivary gland injury using MR sialography. AJNR Am J Neuroradiol 2009;30(1):53–8.

27. Anjos DA, Etchebehere EC, Santos AO, et al. Normal values of [99mTc]pertechnetate uptake and excretion fraction by major salivary glands. Nucl Med Commun 2006;27(4):395–403.

28. Firat F, Cermik TF, Sarikaya A, et al. Effects of gender and age on the quantitative parameters of [99mTc] pertechnetate salivary gland scintigraphy in normal subjects. Nucl Med Commun 2006;27(5):447–53.

29. van den Akker HP, Sokole EB. Sequential scintigraphy of the salivary glands with special reference to the oral activity. Int J Oral Surg 1974;3(5): 321–5.

30. Nishi M, Mimura T, Marutani K, et al. Evaluation of submandibular gland function by sialo-scintigraphy following sialolithectomy. J Oral Maxillofac Surg 1987;45(7):567–71.

31. Yoshimura Y, Morishita T, Sugihara T. Salivary gland function after sialolithiasis: scintigraphic examination of submandibular glands with 99mTc-pertechnetate. J Oral Maxillofac Surg 1989;47(7):704–10 [discussion: 710–1].

32. Seifert G, Donath K. Zur Pathogenese des Küttner-Tumors der Submandibularis - Analyse von 349 Fällen mit chronischer Sialadenitis der Submandibularis. HNO 1977;25(3):81–92 [German].

33. Küttner H. Über entzündliche Tumoren der Submaxillar-Speicheldrüse. Bruns'Beitr Klin Chir 1896;15:815–28 [German].

34. Ahuja AT, Richards PS, Wong KT, et al. Kuttner tumour (chronic sclerosing sialadenitis) of the submandibular gland: sonographic appearances. Ultrasound Med Biol 2003;29(7):913–9.

35. Schwerk WB, Schroeder HG, Eichhorn T. Hochauflösende Real-Time-Sonographie bei Speicheldrüsenerkrankungen. I: Entzündliche Erkrankungen. HNO 1985;33(11):505–10 [German].

36. Rubaltelli L, Sponga T, Candiani F, et al. Infantile recurrent sialectatic parotitis: the role of sonography and sialography in diagnosis and follow-up. Br J Radiol 1987;60(720):1211–4.

37. Koch M, Iro H, Zenk J. Role of sialoscopy in the treatment of Stensen's duct strictures. Ann Otol Rhinol Laryngol 2008;117(4):271–8.

38. Zenk J, Constantinidis J, Al-Kadah B, et al. Transoral removal of submandibular stones. Arch Otolaryngol Head Neck Surg 2001;127(4):432–6.

39. Becker M, Marchal F, Becker CD, et al. Sialolithiasis and salivary ductal stenosis: diagnostic accuracy of MR sialography with a three-dimensional extended-phase conjugate-symmetry rapid spin-echo sequence. Radiology 2000;217(2):347–58.

40. Geisthoff UW, Lehnert BK, Verse T. Ultrasound-guided mechanical intraductal stone fragmentation and removal for sialolithiasis: a new technique. Surg Endosc 2006;20(4):690–4.

41. Iro H, Zenk J, Waldfahrer F, et al. Extracorporeal shock wave lithotripsy of parotid stones. Results of a prospective clinical trial. Ann Otol Rhinol Laryngol 1998;107(10 Pt 1):860–4.

42. Zenk J, Bozzato A, Winter M, et al. Extracorporeal shock wave lithotripsy of submandibular stones: evaluation after 10 years. Ann Otol Rhinol Laryngol 2004;113(5):378–83.

43. Ottaviani F, Capaccio P, Rivolta R, et al. Salivary gland stones: US evaluation in shock wave lithotripsy. Radiology 1997;204(2):437–41.

44. Sittel C, Jungehulsing M, Fischbach R. High-resolution magnetic resonance imaging of recurrent pneumoparotitis. Ann Otol Rhinol Laryngol 1999;108(8): 816–8.

45. Shiboski CH, Hodgson TA, Ship JA, et al. Management of salivary hypofunction during and after radiotherapy. Oral Surg Oral Med Oral Pathol Oral Radiol Endod 2007;103(Suppl):S66 e1–19.

46. Nomayr A, Lell M, Sweeney R, et al. MRI appearance of radiation-induced changes of normal cervical tissues. Eur Radiol 2001;11(9):1807–17.

47. Nishiyama S, Miyawaki S, Yoshinaga Y. A study to standardize quantitative evaluation of parotid gland scintigraphy in patients with Sjögren's syndrome. J Rheumatol 2006;33(12):2470–4.

48. Rubin P, Holt JF. Secretory sialography in diseases of the major salivary glands. Am J Roentgenol Radium Ther Nucl Med 1957;77(4):575–98.

49. Fischer T, Muhler M, Beyersdorff D, et al. Einsatz moderner Ultraschallverfahren in der Diagnostik der Speicheldrüsensarkoidose (Heerfordt-Syndrom). HNO 2003;51(5):394–9 [German].

50. Robson CD, Hazra R, Barnes PD, et al. Nontuberculous mycobacterial infection of the head and neck in immunocompetent children: CT and MR findings. AJNR Am J Neuroradiol 1999;20(10):1829–35.

51. Rabinov K, Weber AL. Radiology of the salivary glands. Boston (MA): G.K.Hall; 1984.

52. Bozzato A, Burger P, Zenk J, et al. Salivary gland biometry in female patients with eating disorders. Eur Arch Otorhinolaryngol 2008; 265(9):1095–102.

Diagnosis and Management of Salivary Gland Infections

Eric R. Carlson, DMD, MD, FACS

KEYWORDS

- Sialadenitis • Sialolithiasis • Acute bacterial parotitis
- Acute bacterial submandibular sialadenitis
- Sialoendoscopy

Salivary gland infections, generically referred to as sialadenitis, have numerous clinical and radiographic presentations and predisposing factors, and are capable of affecting any of the major or minor glands. The earliest case of acute bacterial sialadenitis was reported in 1828 and involved a 71-year-old man with a parotid infection that progressed to gangrene.[1] The significance of parotitis increased in 1881 when President James Garfield reportedly died from an acute parotitis following abdominal surgery related to an assassination attempt. While many accounts refer to his death as an assassination, in fact, President Garfield perished 11 weeks after being shot twice and recovering from his injuries in the White House. Garfield's condition weakened under the oppressive heat and humidity of the Washington summer, undoubtedly suffering complications of dehydration. While reviews of his life and death do not document a specific diagnosis of parotitis, modern day accounts in the medical literature certainly point to this complication.[1]

Sialadenitis may be classified as acute or chronic, and may be of bacterial, viral, fungal, mycobacterial, parasitic, or of an immunologically mediated etiology (**Box 1**). This notwithstanding, bacterial infections of the submandibular and parotid glands are the most common cause and sites of sialadenitis. A number of factors may predispose patients to sialadenitis, typically those that are modifiable, nonmodifiable, or relatively nonmodifiable[2] (**Box 2**). In particular, dehydration with or without recent surgery and anesthesia, medications with known anticholinergic properties, and the presence of a sialolith are well recognized, reversible predisposing features that may create salivary stasis and contribute to sialadenitis. It is evident that the clinician should reverse such conditions during the acute phase of the sialadenitis to prevent spread of infection or the development of a chronic sialadenitis. Consequently, these predisposing features are distinctly modifiable. At the other end of the spectrum, advanced age represents a nonmodifiable predisposing feature, likely due to hyposalivation. Formerly, it was believed that hyposalivation in elderly patients was inevitably due to the aging process, presumably due to loss of functioning acini. It is now recognized, however, that reductions in salivary flow associated with age are modest and probably not associated with a reduction in salivary function. Rather, hyposalivation in the elderly is probably the cumulative result of other factors such as medications.[3] Between these two extremes are the relatively nonmodifiable predisposing features represented by chronic medical diagnoses that may be palliated with resultant diminution in existing sialadenitis. It is important to provide medical therapy of the underlying condition that has predisposed the patient to the sialadenitis, while also directly treating the infection. Rigid glycemic control of diabetes and the use of protease inhibitors in HIV/AIDS are two good examples where medical therapy for these diagnoses can result in decreased salivary symptoms associated with sialadenitis.

Department of Oral and Maxillofacial Surgery, University of Tennessee Graduate School of Medicine, University of Tennessee Cancer Institute, Suite 335, 1930 Alcoa Highway, Knoxville, TN 37920, USA
E-mail address: ecarlson@mc.utmck.edu

Oral Maxillofacial Surg Clin N Am 21 (2009) 293–312
doi:10.1016/j.coms.2009.04.004

oralmaxsurgery.theclinics.com

Box 1
Salivary gland infections

Bacterial infections

    Acute allergic sialadenitis

    Acute bacterial parotitis

    Chronic bacterial parotitis

    Chronic recurrent juvenile parotitis

    Acute suppurative submandibular sialadenitis

    Chronic recurrent submandibular sialadenitis

Viral infections

    Cytomegalovirus

    HIV/AIDS

    Mumps

Fungal infections

Mycobacterial infections

    Atypical mycobacteria

    Tuberculosis

Parasitic infections

    Hydatid disease

Autoimmune-related infections

    Sarcoidosis

    Sjögren syndrome

    Systemic lupus erythematosus

Box 2
Predisposing features associated with infections of the salivary glands

Nonmodifiable predisposing features

Elderly age

Relatively nonmodifiable predisposing features

Anorexia nervosa or bulimia

Congestive heart failure

Cushing's disease

Cystic fibrosis

Diabetes mellitus

HIV/AIDS

Hepatic failure

Radiation therapy where cytoprotective agents were not administered

Renal failure

Modifiable predisposing features

Dehydration

Malnutrition

Medications

    Antihistamines

    Anticholinergics

    Antisialogogues

    Barbiturates

    Chemotherapy drugs

    Diuretics

    Phenothiazines

    Tricyclic antidepressants

Oral infection

Recent surgery and anesthesia

Sialolithiasis

Observation of such medical therapy in these patients, or reinstitution of medications in noncompliant patients will properly address these relatively modifiable predisposing features. Once again, it is incumbent on the clinician to intervene in a timely fashion to lessen the likelihood of the development of chronic sialadenitis. To this end, it is evident that most of the predisposing features of sialadenitis have some degree of reversibility. Early patient presentation and identification of the predisposing feature or features represents an opportunity to predict the reversible nature of the sialadenitis with the avoidance of chronic disease. In addition, following resolution of the sialadenitis associated with a chronic medical condition, measures should be taken to provide proper control of that medical condition. Patient education and compliance with prescribed medications for their underlying condition are paramount in reducing the chances for a recurrence of the acute sialadenitis or for the progression of the acute sialadenitis to a chronic sialadenitis.

INITIAL EVALUATION

The initial evaluation of a patient with a salivary gland swelling must begin with a comprehensive history and physical examination (**Fig. 1**). Several issues are important to address in this initial evaluation, including whether the examination is occurring in an inpatient or outpatient setting; the specific symptoms experienced by the patient; the chronicity of those symptoms; the presence of modifiable, nonmodifiable or relatively nonmodifiable predisposing features; the performance of a physical examination with evaluation of plain radiographs such as a panoramic radiograph and

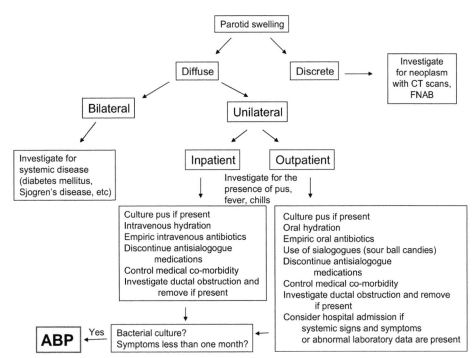

Fig. 1. The algorithm for diagnosis and initial treatment of a generic parotid swelling. Since many cases of siala-denitis are managed conservatively initially, and without an imaging study, the history and physical examination must disclose the presence of a discrete mass to diagnose neoplastic disease in a timely fashion. Failure to do so may delay treatment for a malignant salivary gland tumor.

occlusal radiograph; and, finally, the decision whether sophisticated imaging studies are required to assist in the diagnosis and treatment planning. Additionally, if outpatients are being evaluated, it must be determined if they require admission to the hospital for the administration of intravenous antibiotics and oversight of medical comorbidity.

The setting in which this initial evaluation occurs provides valuable information as to the cause of the sialadenitis. Briefly, the microbiologic cause and treatment of a community-acquired sialadenitis is different from that of a hospital-acquired sialadenitis. As such, the clinician may begin to glean important information as to the cause of the siala-denitis based on the setting in which he or she is examining the patient. Generally, gram-positive organisms are more commonly encountered in community-acquired infections while gram-negative organisms are more commonly encountered in hospital-acquired infections.

Symptoms being experienced by patients with salivary gland enlargement may divulge their disease state and qualify its magnitude. The presence of a painful swelling, particularly prandial pain, or pain during eating, is telling of a diagnosis of sialolithiasis. It is not pathognomonic of a diagnosis of sialolithiasis, however, as sialadenitis

unrelated to sialolithiasis may present in such a fashion. The patient's perception of the expression of pus from the salivary duct should be ascertained during the history. Clearly, the greater the magnitude of purulent infection noted on physical examination, the greater the likelihood that admission to the hospital and incision and drainage will be necessary. In addition, the presence of a significant volume of pus at the opening of a salivary duct may point to the value of obtaining special imaging studies for proper patient management.

The designation of chronicity is important from the standpoint of possible surgical intervention and prognosis. An acute sialadenitis may be diagnosed when symptoms have existed for less than 1 month, while a chronic sialadenitis is considered when symptoms are of greater than 1 month in duration.[2] A more elaborate, yet qualitative description defines an acute sialadenitis in a patient with a previously normal gland, with a sudden onset of diffuse and ill-defined swelling of the entire gland with pain, and possibly erythema and purulence at the papilla of the duct.[4] A chronic sialadenitis may show the gradual development of diffuse swelling of the gland, or a discrete well-defined mass of the gland that may be nonpainful.[4] It should be clear that the latter definition may be confused with a salivary neoplasm, such that special imaging studies may be warranted to assist in the diagnosis. While obtaining the patient's past medical history, it is important to focus on medications taken by the patient that might predispose that patient to xerostomia, thereby encouraging bacterial infection of the salivary glands. A thorough history also serves the purpose of identifying other modifiable and relatively nonmodifiable predisposing features of salivary gland infections.

The physical examination is performed in a focused fashion in the head and neck region in a patient suspected of having a sialadenitis. Specifically, the salivary glands are examined carefully for the presence of asymmetries, warmth, erythema, and swelling. One of the most important aspects of this examination is to consider the presence of a discrete mass that may be indicative or suggestive of a neoplastic process. Specifically, it is important to ascertain the existence of a discrete mass to diagnose a neoplastic process of the salivary glands in a timely fashion. In general terms, an acute inflammatory process of the salivary glands is manifest by diffuse swelling and tenderness while a neoplastic process will show a discrete mass on examination (**Fig. 2**).

Obtaining a screening panoramic radiograph is essential in a patient for whom a clinical diagnosis of sialadenitis of the parotid gland or submandibular gland has been made. The purpose of obtaining such a radiograph is to ascertain the presence of a sialolith. Obtaining an occlusal radiograph may be of value when investigating the presence of a sialolith of the floor of mouth. In addition, obtaining CT scans may be valuable when screening plain films do not identify a sialolith (**Fig. 3**). Sialolithiasis most commonly presents with painful swelling, although a painless swelling or isolated glandular pain may occur. Lustmann and colleagues[5] found swelling to be present in 94% of their 245 cases of sialolithiasis, with pain occurring in 65.2%, the presence of purulence in 15.5%, and complete lack of symptoms in 2.4% of their cases. Regardless of the exact symptom complex associated with sialolithiasis, the fact remains that sialolithiasis and sialadenitis may mimic one another such that a screening radiograph is required to distinguish these two processes. Clearly, the identification of a sialolith will direct care accordingly. However, it must be kept in mind that 80% of submandibular stones are radio-opaque, 40% of parotid stones are radio-opaque, and 20% of sublingual gland stones are radio-opaque;[6] thus, 20% of submandibular stones, 60% of parotid stones, and 80% of sublingual stones will not appear on a screening panoramic radiograph. In such cases, it is likely that an inaccurate, isolated diagnosis of sialadenitis will be made initially with the development of refractory disease and potentially the ultimate removal of the salivary gland. At the time of gland removal, the stone will be identified and the diagnosis of sialolithiasis will be realized (**Fig. 4**).

Finally, the surgeon may wish to obtain special imaging studies, such as CT scans or MRIs, when dealing with a patient with salivary gland swelling. Three circumstances dictate obtaining such a study. The first is when a discrete mass is detected that is suggestive of a neoplastic process. This study permits anatomic delineation of the neoplasm and allows for the planning of a precision tumor surgery. This statement is particularly true when planning parotid surgery.[7] Second, CT or MRI may be indicated when managing a refractory sialadenitis in preparation for surgery. Finally, the presence of significant purulence at the salivary duct may be indicative of an abscess requiring drainage. Obtaining an imaging study will assist the surgeon in determining if an incision and drainage procedure is emergently indicated, and where the drainage should be directed.

While primary causes of sialadenitis are microbiologically or immunologically based, there are secondary causes of sialadenitis worth mentioning. Trauma, in particular, is worth considering as far as the diagnosis of sialadenitis is concerned. Specifically, there are two circumstances in which trauma may be of significance. The first is the patient who has sustained penetrating facial trauma with potential involvement of Stenson's duct whereby primary closure may result in intentional or inadvertent ligation of the duct. Inadvertent ligation of the salivary duct will create an obstructive sialadenitis. To avoid such a problem, the primary trauma surgeon must consider the anatomic location of the salivary duct and provide reconstruction of that duct as necessary. The integrity of the duct may be assessed with a variety of sterile media (**Fig. 5**). This example is therefore preventive in nature. The second example of trauma-induced sialadenitis is where inadvertent ligation of the duct has occurred related to a biopsy of a lesion in proximity of the salivary gland duct. The patient therefore presents with salivary gland swelling and pain, and a diagnosis of obstructive sialadenitis is made following a surgical procedure. Under these circumstances, the clinician must correlate the history and physical examination, with consideration for the removal of the affected salivary gland (**Fig. 6**). This example, therefore, is interventional in nature.

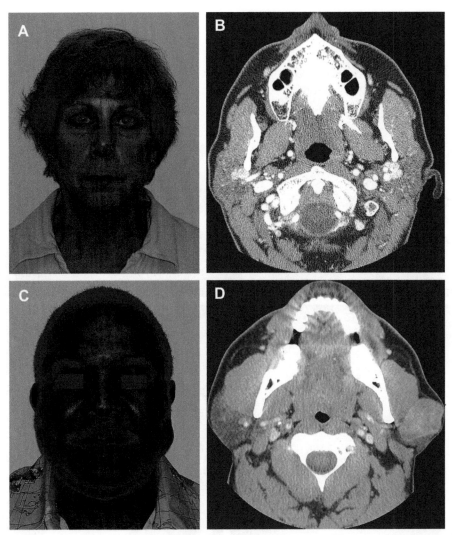

Fig. 2. Two patients with parotid swellings of different etiologies. (*A*) 55-year-old woman with a 10-year history of intermittent left parotid swelling and pain. Diffuse swelling was appreciated on physical examination and CT scans (*B*) did not reveal a concerning mass within the left parotid gland. A clinical and radiographic diagnosis of chronic recurrent bacterial parotitis was offered. This presentation is very different from a 52-year-old man with a 4-year history of a left parotid swelling (*C*). In this case, a discrete mass is visualized and palpated. CT scans confirmed the presence of a discrete mass (*D*). This patient underwent a superficial parotidectomy and a pleomorphic adenoma was diagnosed. The history and physical examination of a patient with a parotid swelling should initiate the process of distinguishing an inflammatory process from a neoplastic process.

BACTERIAL SALIVARY GLAND INFECTIONS
Acute Bacterial Parotitis

Before the modern surgical era, acute bacterial parotitis (ABP) was a feared complication of major surgical procedures and carried a mortality rate as high as 50%.[8] Inadequate postoperative resuscitation with crystalloid solutions, including the development of decreased salivary flow and xerostomia, was common. In addition, the reduction of salivary stimulation due to the patient not eating in the early postoperative period predisposed patients to acute bacterial parotitis, with an

incidence of about 0.1%.[9] In addition, the lack of available antistaphylococcal antibiotics led to acute bacterial parotitis. Specifically, it has been calculated that the incidence of acute bacterial parotitis was 3.68 cases per 10,000 operations (0.0368%) in the preantibiotic era compared to 0.173 cases per 10,000 operations (0.00173%) in the postantibiotic era.[10]

The bacterial flora of the oral cavity has noticeably changed over the last several decades that have changed the microbiological profile of acute bacterial parotitis. This has occurred for three

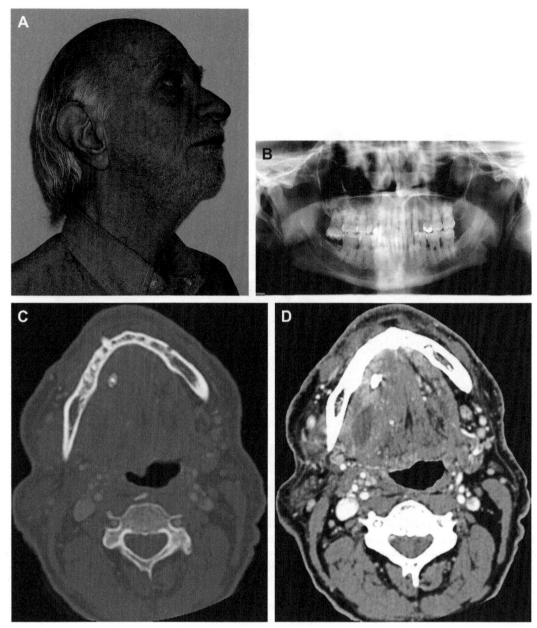

Fig. 3. A 73-year-old man with an acute onset of right submandibular swelling and pain (*A*). A screening panoramic radiograph did not identify the presence of a sialolith (*B*). Owing to the large amount of pus that was expressed from Wharton's duct, CT scans were obtained that identified an abscess in the submandibular gland and a sialolith in the extraglandular duct (*C, D*). The patient was admitted to the hospital for the administration of intravenous antibiotics as well as intravenous fluid hydration. The right submandibular gland was removed along with extraglandular sialolithotomy several weeks later (*E, F*). He was noted to be well healed and without pain at 6-months postoperatively (*G*).

reasons. The first is the increased incidence of nosocomial and opportunistic infections in patients who are immunocompromised and those critically ill patients in hospital ICUs whose mouths became colonized with organisms rarely previously found in the oral cavity. Second, improved techniques in recovery of microorganisms have permitted the identification of anaerobes that were previously difficult to culture in microbiology laboratories. Third, the routine and nonscientific use of oral antibiotics in the community has resulted in the occupation of organisms in the oral cavity not previously seen and the development of antibiotic resistance by organisms commonly seen.

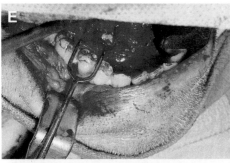

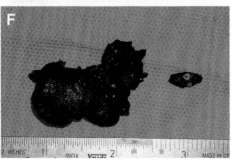

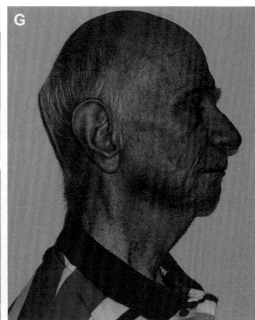

Fig. 3. (*continued*)

Acute bacterial parotitis has two well-recognized variants; hospital-acquired form and community-acquired form. Retrograde infection of the parotid gland is well-accepted as the major cause of ABP. Diminished salivary flow resulting from inadequate intravascular volume related to sepsis, acute illness, or the postoperative state may result in diminished flushing action of saliva as it passes through Stenson's duct. When salivary secretions are adequate in their volume, bacteria are noted at the duct papillae but not within the duct, while depressed salivary secretions result in the presence of bacteria at the papillae and in the duct.[11] Fibronectin is noted to exist in high concentrations within parotid saliva in a healthy state, thereby encouraging the adherence of *Streptococcus* species and *Staphylococcus aureus* at the orifice of Stenson's duct. In an unhealthy host fibronectin is deficient, which promotes the adherence of *Pseudomonas* and *Escherichia coli*.[11] This observation helps to explain the presence of a gram-positive sialadenitis in the presence of dehydration and gram-negative sialadenitis in the immunocompromised patients.[12] It is primarily the health of the patient, therefore, that determines which bacteria preferentially infect the parotid gland in a retrograde fashion. Hospital-acquired ABP shows cultures of *Staphylococcus aureus* in over 50% of cases, and methicillin resistance should be investigated in the microbiology laboratory. Intensive care unit patients may also show infection with *Eikenella*

corrodens, Escherichia coli, Fusobacterium, Haemophilus influenzae, Klebsiella, Prevotella, Proteus, and *Pseudomonas* species. From the standpoint of timing, most cases of ABP occur between postoperative days 5 and 7, although it has been diagnosed from 1 to 15 weeks following surgery.[1]

Community-acquired ABP is more commonly diagnosed than hospital-acquired ABP, and will be identified in outpatient health care settings. This variant of ABP is typically associated with *Staphylococcal* and *Streptococcal* species. Factors of significance in community-acquired ABP include medications that decrease salivary flow, cheek biting, medical conditions such as diabetes, malnutrition, and dehydration from gastrointestinal disorders associated with loss of intravascular volume such as diarrhea and vomiting.

Diagnosis and treatment of ABP

Paramount to the diagnosis and treatment of pathology of the head and neck, a comprehensive history and physical examination is central in the diagnosis and treatment of ABP (**Fig. 7**). A history of antisialogogue medications, malnutrition, diabetes mellitus or other systemic diseases, dehydration, or recent surgery are important historical issues to divulge. Males seem to be more commonly afflicted with ABP, and the average age at presentation is 60 years. The right gland is more commonly affected when the disease is unilateral.[2] Classic symptoms include an abrupt

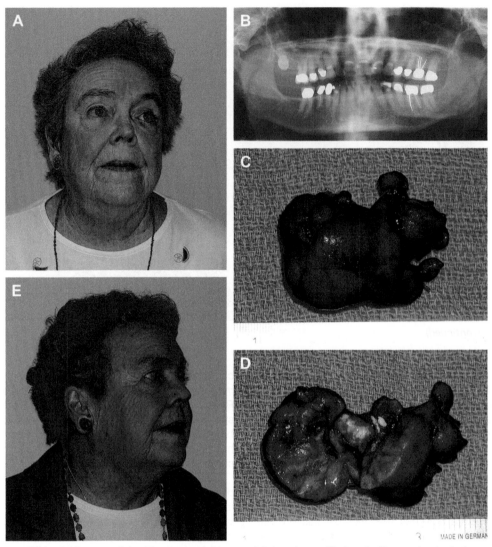

Fig. 4. An 83-year-old woman (*A*) with a 6-month history of right submandibular swelling and pain during eating. A clinical diagnosis of chronic submandibular sialadenitis was made and a screening panoramic radiograph (*B*) did not reveal the presence of a sialolith. The patient underwent right submandibular gland excision (*C*). The specimen was bivalved on the back table in the operating room and a sialolith was noted (*D*). The patient's neck incision is well healed 6 months postoperatively (*E*).

history of painful swelling of the parotid region, especially when eating. If Stenson's duct is patent, palpation of the gland may result in the expression of pus. Under such circumstances, the pus should be sampled in a sterile fashion and submitted for culture and sensitivity. The initial consultation appointment should investigate the presence of systemic signs and symptoms including fever and chills. Concerning historical and physical findings should result in the ordering of a complete blood count and a basic metabolic panel. A leukocytosis and signs consistent with dehydration, including hypernatremia and an elevated blood urea nitrogen, may be disclosed. This information

may be valuable in making a decision whether the patient with ABP should be admitted to the hospital for intravenous hydration and the administration of intravenous antibiotics. An admission to the hospital is also an opportunity to control medical comorbidity. As stated earlier, a screening panoramic radiograph should be obtained that may reveal the presence of a sialolith responsible for an obstructive parotid sialadenitis.

For the most part, patients with acute sialadenitis may be managed empirically. This statement applies specifically to those patients with minimal symptoms related to a clinical diagnosis of sialadenitis. For example, a patient with a swollen

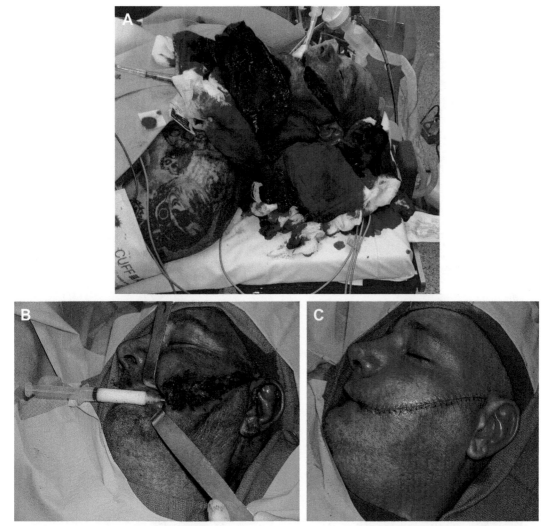

Fig. 5. A 46-year-old man who sustained a knife wound of the left face that has resulted in a significant loss of blood due to transaction of branches of the facial artery and vein (*A*). Inherent in the immediate operative procedure is ligation of transected blood vessels as well as exploration of the left Stenson's duct to determine the integrity of the duct. The anatomic location of Stenson's duct can be predicted by an imaginary line connecting the tragus of the ear to the midphiltral region of the upper lip. In this case, the distal end of Stenson's duct was cannulated and sterile milk was injected (*B*). The white color of the milk would permit the identification of this liquid in the wound if injury to the duct existed. No milk was identified in the wound such that anatomic closure of the wound was accomplished without concern for the salivary duct (*C*).

and tender submandibular or parotid gland with minimal or no exudate noted at their duct and with diffuse swelling rather than a discrete mass can probably be initially managed with a regimen of digital massage, oral antibiotics, the use of heat, proper hydration, and sialogogues (sour ball candies) on an out-patient basis (see **Fig. 7**). As previously noted, a screening panoramic radiograph is routinely indicated to rule out the possibility of a sialolith responsible for an obstructive sialadenitis. If a sialolith is identified in an extraglandular site, its removal should be promptly

performed after which time the patient's symptoms should be monitored for improvement. In general terms, a stone that is able to be palpated transorally can be removed without having to sacrifice the salivary gland. Under such circumstances, removal of the salivary gland is reserved for patients who develop a refractory sialadenitis.

A clinical diagnosis of ABP without the clinical presence of pus and without systemic signs and symptoms represents an opportunity for outpatient management without the need to obtain special imaging studies. Exploration of Stenson's

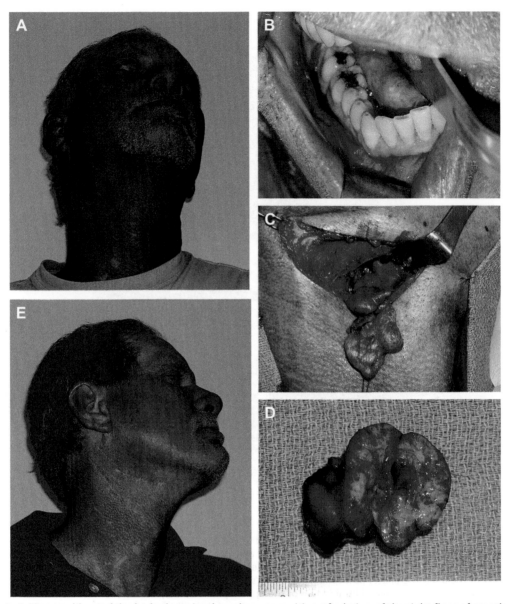

Fig. 6. A 53-year-old man (*A*) who had previously undergone excision of a lesion of the right floor of mouth. He described right submandibular prandial pain shortly thereafter. No expression of saliva was appreciated at the opening of Wharton's duct, and scar tissue was noted in the right floor of mouth in the region of Wharton's duct (*B*). A diagnosis of obstructive submandibular sialadenitis was made and the patient was subjected to right submandibular excision. Dissection of the distal duct in the region of the right lingual nerve resulted in the expression of obstructed mucous (*C*). The bivalved specimen (*D*) showed scar. The patient exhibited no pain, as noted in his 6-month postoperative appearance (*E*).

duct with probes during the acute setting of ABP is probably contraindicated because of the fear of encouraging the progression of the infection proximally in the gland.[2] Initial measures for management of ABP are similar for hospital-acquired and community-acquired infections (see **Fig. 1**). It is appropriate to provide a sample of purulent exudate at Stenson's duct for culture and sensitivity and to place patients on empiric antibiotics. Intravenous antibiotics are used for inpatients and oral antibiotics are typically prescribed for outpatients. It is important to determine if outpatients have systemic signs and symptoms, or an ABP of significant magnitude, under which circumstances an inpatient admission might be warranted for the administration of intravenous

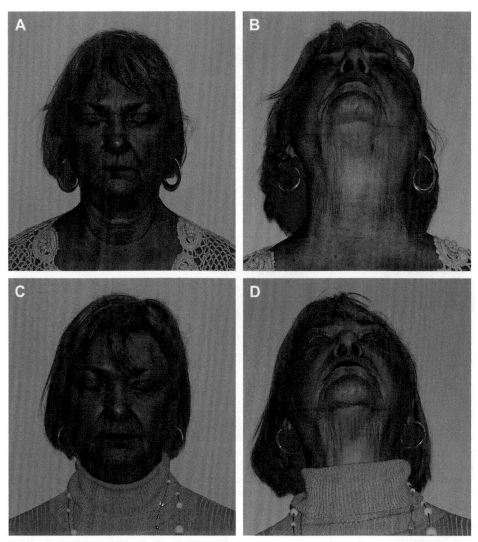

Fig. 7. A 55-year-old woman with an acute history of pain and swelling in the left parotid gland (*A, B*). Physical examination did not reveal the presence of pus at left Stenson's duct. The patient was taking tolterodine, an anticholinergic medication, for overactive bladder with incontinence. Initial therapy consisted of discontinuation of the tolterodine, and institution of sourball candy use, oral antibiotics, digital massage of the left parotid gland, and the application of heat to the left face. Two weeks later, the patient was asymptomatic and the swelling had resolved (*C, D*). Her ABP has not recurred. (*Reprinted from* Carlson ER, Ord RA, editors. Textbook and color atlas of salivary gland pathology. Diagnosis and management. Wiley-Blackwell, Ames [IA]; 2008. p. 68; with permission.)

antibiotics (**Fig. 8**) and possible drainage of a parotid abscess. Patients presenting with an ABP with systemic signs and symptoms clearly require imaging with CT scans or MRI scans to determine the presence of a parotid abscess. The institution of conservative measures should be monitored very closely in inpatients and outpatients for 48 to 72 hours, after which time follow-up must occur (**Fig. 9**). Clinical deterioration, as noted by increased parotid swelling and pain, increased volume of pus, or an increase in the white blood cell count, should be addressed by obtaining an imaging study with likely plans for incision and drainage. The progression of acute bacterial parotitis to chronic bacterial parotitis (CBP) occurs in three settings. The first occurs in which the patient develops an ABP but defers evaluation such that the condition is permitted to enter a chronic state beyond 1 month. The second setting occurs in the face of a timely managed ABP that develops refractory sialadenitis. Third, an untreated parotitis can develop remitting and relapsing disease in which latent infection exists despite clinical evidence of resolution of the disease.

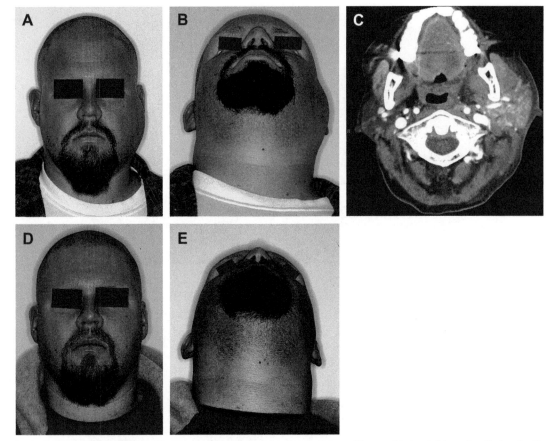

Fig. 8. A 37-year-old man (*A, B*) with a 3-day history of left parotid swelling and intractable pain. Owing to the magnitude of the patient's symptoms, he was admitted to the hospital for the administration of intravenous antibiotics. CT scans were obtained (*C*) that showed signs consistent with parotitis, but without evidence of a sialolith or abscess. His parotid swelling resolved as noted at two weeks following discharge from the hospital (*D, E*).

Chronic Bacterial Parotitis (Chronic Recurrent Parotitis)

CBP, also known as chronic recurrent parotitis, is a nonspecific sialadenitis that is characterized by unilateral or bilateral swellings with either periodic episodic relapsing and remitting swellings of the parotid gland, or persistent symptoms of the involved gland.[13] The etiology of this condition is probably multifactorial; however, a common factor is salivary stasis with a predisposition to infection.[14] Inflammation is thought to cause multifocal wall irregularities which propagate into stricture formation.[13] Typically, CBP begins with an episode of ABP. CBP should not be confused with secondary infections that occur in the presence of a sialolith or Sjögren's syndrome. Sialoliths cause obstruction with resultant salivary stasis, not unlike CBP. The sialolith, however, is the known primary factor that acts to create the secondary parotitis. The same is true for Sjögren's syndrome patients who have a marked decrease

in salivary production that encourages the development of an ascending infection. Again, Sjogren's syndrome is the primary pathologic process on which a parotitis secondarily occurs. Like sialolithiasis and Sjögren's syndrome, CBP is a primary pathologic process, the result of which is decreased salivary production.

Clinically, CBP occurs with a sudden onset of diffuse parotid swelling, typically unilateral but occasionally bilateral, with varying degrees of discomfort. There is no known relationship with meals or seasons, suggesting no obstructive or allergic phenomena.[15] The swelling may persist for days, weeks, or months, and an associated low-grade fever is common. The swellings resolve and are associated with periods of clinical quiescence ranging from weeks to years. Pus is not typically observed, but rather a material referred to as mucopus is produced that serves to obstruct the salivary duct lumen leading to a condition that favors further bacterial growth and stasis.[13,16] Baurmash[15] disputed the utility of this term, and

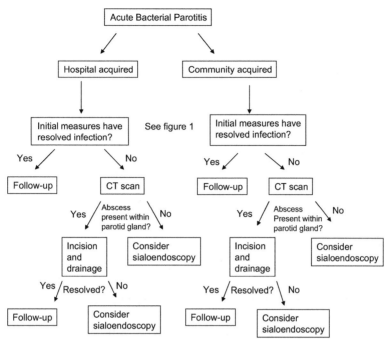

Fig. 9. The follow-up algorithm for patients diagnosed with ABP. This algorithm is followed after the initial protocol outlined in **Fig. 1**.

investigated the true nature of the precipitant within the ductal system. If the presence of pus is unequivocally present for several days, the clinician should consider the possibility of an acute suppurative parotitis superimposed on the CBP and the patient should be treated accordingly.

Classically, two forms of CBP have been described, including adult and juvenile forms. The adult form has been associated with *Staphylococcus aureus* infection, whereas *Streptococcus viridans* is the major pathogenic bacteria in the juvenile form, and children between the ages of 3 and 6 years of age are affected, with males more commonly affected. The disease process may resolve spontaneously at puberty with functional recovery of the parotid gland.[12] See the article on pediatric salivary gland infections elsewhere in this issue.

Diagnosis and treatment of chronic bacterial parotitis

History and physical examination will provide valuable information and several radiographic studies will assist in the diagnosis of CBP. As with ABP, a patient suspected of having a diagnosis of CBP should undergo a screening panoramic radiograph. This film will provide initial information as to whether a sialolith is present. To clearly depict the ductal system of the parotid gland with a radiographic technique, sialographic imaging with a water-soluble contrast medium has been well studied.[13] Chronic parotitis starts

with a punctate sialectasis and dilatation of the peripheral ducts. These dilatations and strictures create a "sausage-like appearance" as observed on sialographic imaging.[13] MRI has been considered the gold standard method for imaging soft tissue pathology, including infections. Its sensitivity exceeds that of CT in this field.[13] Another highly sensitive method is the sialo-MRI, which shows the salivary parenchymal tissues with great accuracy. The sialo-MRI is an imaging technique that is performed without the injection of contrast medium and is considered a noninvasive, painless, and safe technique. Because this study is dependent on salivary flow as the contrast medium, diminished salivary flow will result in an impaired examination.[17]

Treatment of CBP (**Fig. 10**) surrounds two important elements of therapy. The first involves reduction or elimination of inflammation in the gland. Short-term corticosteroids are used to accomplish this goal. Baurmash[15] recommended a tapering schedule of dexamethasone, beginning with 0.75 mg orally, four times daily for 3 days, followed by 0.75 mg orally three times daily for 3 days, followed by 0.75 mg orally twice daily for three days, and finally one-half tablet twice daily for 3 days. Unless an acute infection is superimposed on the pre-existing CBP, antibiotics will not be effective in treating CBP.

The second goal of therapy is to clear the precipitated serum proteins within the intraductal system.

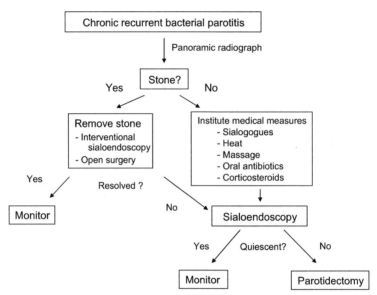

Fig. 10. Algorithm for management of chronic recurrent bacterial parotitis.

One means to accomplish this goal is to increase salivary production and clearance with sialogogues and warm compresses, which probably still represent the first line of therapy.[13] The most effective means to accomplish this goal is to perform diagnostic and interventional sialoendoscopy (**Fig. 11**). One method of sialoendoscopy is directed to overcome the main pathology of CBP: multiple strictures in the salivary duct. In addition, patients are candidates for interventional treatment who suffer from more than one acute episode per year.[13] Under such circumstances, the sialoendoscope is advanced in the duct until it meets obstruction. The advancement of the scope is performed with continuous normal saline lavage that is highly effective in the visualization of the ductal system, and in dilating the strictures within the duct. The sialoballoon may be utilized to provide further dilatation of the ductal system. A stent may be inserted to assist in preventing redevelopment of strictures over a 4-week period. See the article on sialoendoscopy elsewhere in this issue.

Patients with intractable pain related to CBP may become candidates for facial nerve-sparing, superficial parotidectomy (**Fig. 12**). This procedure is performed with the statistical likelihood of the infection being located in the superficial lobe because of its prominence. Imaging studies are critical to determine the anatomic location of the infection prior to performing surgical therapy.

Chronic Recurrent Juvenile Parotitis

Chronic recurrent parotitis in children is typically noted prior to puberty and occurs as numerous episodes of painful enlargements of the parotid gland. This disease in children is ten times more common than chronic recurrent parotitis in adults.[15] Risk factors for this disease include congenital abnormalities or strictures of Stenson's duct, a history of viral mumps, trauma, or foreign bodies within the duct. Conservative measures, including the use of oral antibiotics, are generally recommended as many cases will resolve prior to the onset of puberty. Spontaneous regeneration of salivary function has been reported.[18]

Acute Bacterial Submandibular Sialadenitis

Acute bacterial submandibular sialadenitis (ABSS) is a community-acquired disease that is less frequently associated with dehydration and an inpatient admission to the hospital than ABP. The most common cause of ABSS is obstruction of Wharton's duct, typically from a sialolith. Sialolithiasis most commonly occurs in the submandibular gland for at least two reasons. The first is that the submandibular gland lies inferior to Wharton's duct such that the flow of saliva travels against the forces of gravity, with the relative development of salivary stasis compared to the parotid gland and other major and minor salivary glands. Sialolithiasis results from the deposition of calcium salts within the ductal system of the salivary gland. These stones are primarily comprised of calcium phosphate with traces of magnesium and ammonia with an organic matrix consisting of carbohydrates and amino acids. The relative salivary stasis encourages precipitation of these calcium phosphate salts. Eighty-five

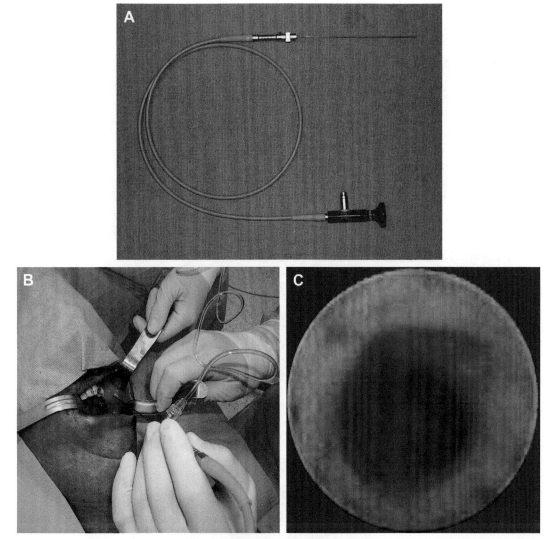

Fig. 11. Instrumentation for a diagnostic sialoendoscopic procedure. The miniature sialoendoscope (Karl Storz Endoscopy-America, Inc., Culver City, California) (*A*) is introduced into Stenson's duct (*B*). Under the pressure of normal saline irrigation, an image of the duct is appreciated (*C*). The mere irrigation of the duct may be therapeutic in the case of CBP. (*A and B reprinted from* Carlson ER, Ord RA, editors. Textbook and color atlas of salivary gland pathology. Diagnosis and management. Wiley-Blackwell, Ames [IA]; 2008. p. 76–7; with permission.)

percent of sialoliths occur in the submandibular gland, 10% in the parotid gland, 5% in the sublingual gland, and an insignificant number of stones occur in the minor salivary glands. With regard to the anatomic location of submandibular stones, 75% to 85% are located within Wharton's duct. In theory, the acute bends of Wharton's duct might also predispose the ductal system to the development of sialolithiasis. This concept has been studied by Drage and collegues[19] who examined the sialograms of 61 patients with sialolithiasis, 23 patients with sialadenitis, and a control group of 18 patients. There were no statistical differences in the angle of the genu of the duct in the three groups, suggesting that the difference in the angle of the genu of the submandibular duct was not a significant cause in the formation of sialoliths. The investigators indicated that the length of Wharton's duct could certainly be a significant cause in the development of sialolithiasis. Second, the alkaline nature of submandibular saliva, its viscosity, and its relatively high content of calcium salts predisposes patients to sialolithiasis.

Diagnosis and treatment of acute bacterial submandibular sialadenitis
The clinical presentation of ABSS includes submandibular gland swelling and prandial pain. Purulence

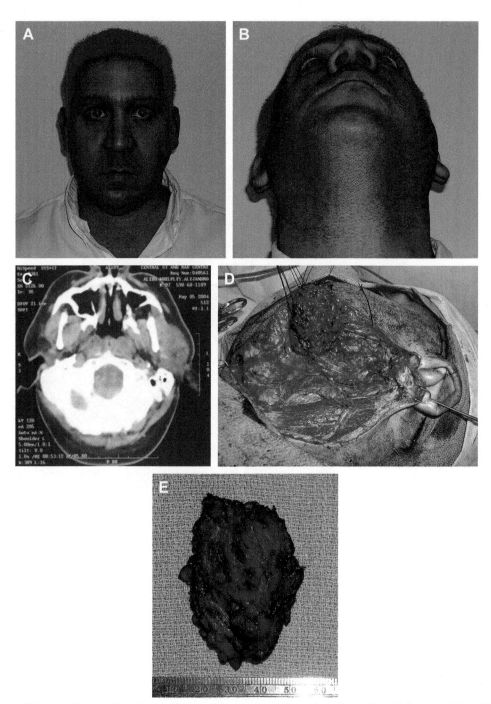

Fig. 12. A-35-year old man with a 2-year history of intractable pain and swelling of the left parotid gland (*A, B*). Computerized scans identified sclerosis of the parotid parenchyma and likely abscess formation within the superficial lobe of the parotid gland (*C*). The patient underwent left superficial parotidectomy with identification and preservation of the facial nerve (*D, E*). At three years postoperatively he is noted without swelling in the parotid region and with a well healed modified Blair incision (*F, G*). (*Reprinted from* Carlson ER, Ord RA, editors. Textbook and color atlas of salivary gland pathology. Diagnosis and management. Wiley-Blackwell, Ames [IA]; 2008. p. 78–9; with permission.)

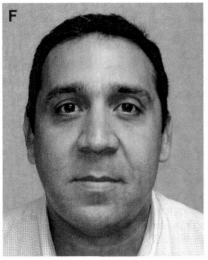
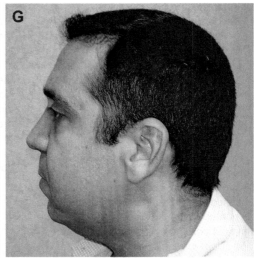

Fig. 12. (*continued*)

may be noted at the opening of Wharton's duct in the floor of mouth. These clinical features permit rapid diagnosis of ABSS. As with a diagnosis of sialadenitis of the parotid gland, a screening panoramic radiograph is indicated for identifying a sialolith, if one is present. Treatment of ABSS involves hydration, avoidance of antisialogogue medications, the use of sialogogues, and removal of a sialolith if one is identified on screening panoramic radiograph. The institution of empiric oral antibiotic therapy is warranted, and may be provided by a broad-spectrum penicillin, first generation cephalosporin, clindamycin, or a macrolide. A more aggressive intervention than that described is rarely necessary, and success may be met with compliance with the regimen without the need to perform a submandibular gland excision.

Chronic Recurrent Submandibular Sialadenitis

Chronic recurrent submandibular sialadenitis usually follows ineffective treatment of ABSS owing to lack of compliance with recommended therapy, the presence of an undiagnosed sialolith, or pre-existing and undiagnosed chronic disease when the patient initially presented with what was believed to represent ABSS. Chronic recurrent submandibular sialadenitis may be initially diagnosed in this state because the patient delayed evaluation and treatment. Chronic recurrent submandibular sialadenitis occurs more commonly than CBP.

Diagnosis and treatment of chronic recurrent submandibular sialadenitis

Patients with chronic recurrent submandibular sialadenitis may report a long history of submandibular gland swelling, infection, and pain. In addition, physical examination will typically show a significantly indurated gland, and occasionally a small gland due to scar contracture. Long-standing disease may produce a tumor-like mass that has been referred to as a Kuttner tumor.[20] While the history and physical examination may be sufficient to give patients this diagnosis, special imaging studies may be obtained that document signs consistent with chronic recurrent submandibular sialadenitis. For example, sialography may demonstrate evidence of sialadenitis and sialectasis, with decreased gland emptying rates indicative of poor gland function.[12] Initial treatment involves empiric antibiotic therapy, sialogogues, and hydration. Ultimately, an indurated and nonfunctional gland will require removal.

Tuberculous Mycobacterial Disease

Infection of the salivary glands with *Mycobacterium tuberculosis* is uncommon but may be seen in older children and adults. Lymph nodes adjacent to salivary glands are much more commonly involved than intraglandular lymph nodes.[21] Intraparenchymal involvement of the parotid gland is usually related to invasion of the gland from disease in the intraglandular lymph nodes.

The presence of mycobacterial disease in the parotid gland in adults is complicated by its clinical resemblance to neoplastic disease. The presence of a discrete mass in such cases requires a fine-needle aspiration biopsy to ascertain the diagnosis. Nonetheless, this may be inconclusive so surgical removal of the gland is usually required to confirm diagnosis.[22] Surgery is technically difficult owing to the fibrotic response to the mycobacterial infection. Once the diagnosis has been established, multi-drug medical therapy is paramount. Obtaining a purified protein derivative skin test and chest radiographs may assist in conclusively arriving at the proper diagnosis.

Nontuberculous Mycobacterial Disease

Atypical mycobacteria may infect the submandibular and parotid glands. These infections are more common in children between 2 and 5 years of age and immunocompromised adult patients. It has been estimated that greater than 92% of mycobacterial cervicofacial infections in children are the result of nontuberculous mycobacteria.[23] The organisms most commonly responsible include *M kansasii, M avium-intracellulare,* and *M scrofulaceum.* The typical clinical presentation is a rapidly enlarging and persistent parotid or neck mass that has failed to resolve with antibiotic therapy.[2] Not uncommonly, a violaceous discoloration develops in the overlying skin. The treatment of choice is surgical removal of the involved salivary gland and draining lymph nodes.

VIRAL SALIVARY GLAND INFECTIONS
Mumps

Mumps is a viral non-suppurative disease that characteristically occurs in the parotid glands in a bilateral fashion. The infection is most commonly caused by a paramyxovirus, a ribonucleic acid virus related to the influenza and parainfluenza virus groups. This notwithstanding, other viruses can cause mumps, including coxsackie A and B, Epstein Barr virus, influenza and parainfluenza, enteric cytopathic human orphan (ECHO) virus, and human immunodeficiency virus (HIV). Epidemic outbreaks generally occur in the spring and winter months. The near routine administration of the measles-mumps-rubella (MMR) vaccination has decreased the incidence of mumps in industrialized nations. The yearly incidence of mumps cases has declined from 76 to 2 cases per 100,000 since the introduction of the live attenuated vaccine in the United States in 1967.[24] The incubation period between exposure to the virus and the development of signs and symptoms is 15-18 days. A prodromal period occurs that lasts 1-2 days and involves fever, chills, headache, and preauricular tenderness. Thereafter, rapid and painful unilateral or bilateral swelling of the parotid glands occurs. The diagnosis is made by demonstrating complement-fixing soluble (S) antibodies to the nucleoprotein core of the virus, which are the earliest antibodies to appear, and therefore associated with active infection. The complement-fixing viral (V) antibodies are against outer surface hemagglutinin and appear later than S antibodies. The V antibodies may persist at low levels for years. Virus may also be isolated in the urine 6 days prior and 13 days following the development of salivary gland symptoms. Complications of mumps include abdominal pain, indicative of mumps pancreatitis, and mumps orchitis that occurs in about 20% of male patients. Mumps thyroiditis, mumps myocarditis, and mumps hepatitis are considered rare complications of mumps infection.[2]

Treatment of mumps is supportive as spontaneous resolution of the disease occurs within 5-10 days following the onset of symptoms. During this time, dietary modifications to minimize glandular activity, proper hydration, and bedrest may be necessary. It may be necessary to provide enteral nutritional tube feeds to patients so as to prevent stimulation of the parotid gland during eating food by mouth.

Human immunodeficiency virus

Human immunodeficiency virus infection (HIV) most commonly affects the parotid gland when it involves the salivary glands. Diffuse involvement of the salivary glands is referred to as HIV associated salivary gland disease (HIV-SGD) and may affect patients with all stages of HIV infection. Patients with HIV-SGD typically present with a history of non-tender swelling of one or more of the salivary glands. These swellings may fluctuate, but are usually persistent and may mimic lymphoepithelial cysts such that imaging studies are indicated to distinguish these processes. Diffuse infiltrative lymphocytosis syndrome (DILS) occurs in patients with HIV and consists of decreased salivary gland function resulting in xerostomia and sicca symptoms. This process is characterized by circulating CD8 lymphocytes that infiltrate organs, particularly the salivary glands. Treatment of HIV-SGD requires the compliant use of antiretroviral medical therapy by patients, the use of sialogogues and possibly corticosteroid medications, and the observation of meticulous oral hygiene.

PARASITIC SALIVARY GLAND INFECTIONS

Hydatid disease of the parotid gland is extremely rare.[25] The primary host of such an infection is the dog that consumes uncooked offal containing hydatid cysts. Under such circumstances, *Echinococcus granulosus* is perpetuated. The parasite, therefore, develops in the dog's intestine and ova are expelled in its feces. The intermediate host, occasionally a human, ingests these eggs. The developing hydatid cyst may remain asymptomatic for many years, and the cyst slowly enlarges. After ingestion, the worm penetrates the wall of the intestine, passing by way of the portal circulation to the liver and occasionally to other organs, though primarily the liver, but possibly to the salivary glands. The diagnosis would be suspected based on the patient's presence in endemic areas, but also based on ultrasonography that will confirm the cystic nature of a swelling. Plain films may show calcification of the cyst wall as curved lines, rings, or spotty calcification in degenerating cysts.[25] The disease is rarely diagnosed preoperatively. Rather, the diagnosis is made based on histopathologic specimens. Nonetheless, it is important not to rupture the cyst intraoperatively because of the possibility of anaphylactic shock. Proper surgical technique and preoperative administration of corticosteroids will minimize this complication.

COLLAGEN SIALADENITIS

Autoimmune disorders, including scleroderma, dermatomyositis, polymyositis, and systemic lupus erythematosus may affect the salivary glands. Owing to the autoimmune nature of these disorders, women are most commonly affected, in the fourth and fifth decades. All of the salivary glands can become involved. The presentation is typically a slowly enlarging salivary gland. The diagnosis is made by identifying the underlying systemic disorder, and salivary chemistry levels will reveal sodium and chloride ion levels that are elevated two to three times over normal levels.[12] The treatment of collagen sialadenitis involves treatment of the underlying systemic disease.

SUMMARY

Salivary gland infections have a diverse set of risk factors, causes, and treatment strategies. Usually, if possible, the goal of management of such infections is to preserve the gland. Medical therapy and minimally invasive surgical therapy are designed to resort to removal of the salivary gland as a final effort in eliminating salivary gland infections. While examining and planning the workup and treatment of a patient with swelling of a salivary gland, it is paramount to consider the likelihood of a neoplasm masquerading as an infection.

REFERENCES

1. McQuone SJ. Acute viral and bacterial infections of the salivary glands. Otolaryngol Clin North Am 1999;32(5):794–811.

2. Carlson ER, Ord RA. Infections of the salivary glands. In: Carlson ER, Ord RA, editors. Textbook and color atlas of salivary gland pathology. Diagnosis and management. Ames (IA): Wiley-Blackwell; 2008. p. 67–89.

3. Neville BW, Damm DD, Allen CM, et al. Salivary gland pathology. In: Neville BW, Damm DD, Allen CM, editors. Oral and maxillofacial pathology. 3rd edition. St. Louis (MO): Saunders Elsevier; 2009. p. 453–506.

4. Marchal F, Bradley PJ. Management of infections of the salivary glands. In: Myers EN, Ferris RL, editors. Salivary gland disorders. Berlin: Springer-Verlag; 2007. p. 169–76.

5. Lustmann J, Regev E, Melamed Y. Sialolithiasis: a survey on 245 patients and a review of the literature. Int J Oral Maxillofac Surg 1990;19:135–8.

6. Miloro M. The surgical management of submandibular gland disease. Atlas Oral Maxillofac Surg Clin North Am 1998;6:29–50.

7. Carlson ER. Parotid tumor. In: Laskin DM, Abubaker AO, editors. Decision making in oral and maxillofacial surgery. Chicago: Quintessence Publishing Co. Inc.; 2007. p. 212–3.

8. Goldberg MH, Bevilacqua RG. Infections of the salivary glands. Oral Maxillofac Surg Clin North Am 1995;3:423–30.

9. Andrews JC, Abemayor E, Alessi DM, et al. Parotitis and facial nerve dysfunction. Arch Otolaryngol Head Neck Surg 1989;115:240–2.

10. Robinson JR. Surgical parotitis, vanishing disease. Surgery 1955;38:703–7.

11. Katz J, Fisher D, Levine S. Bacterial colonization of the parotid duct in xerostomia. Int J Oral Maxillofac Surg 1990;19:7–9.

12. Miloro M, Goldberg MH. Salivary gland infections. In: Topazian RG, Goldberg MH, Hupp JR, editors. Oral and maxillofacial infections. 4th edition. Philadelphia: W.B. Saunders; 2002. p. 279–93.

13. Nahlieli O, Bar T, Shacham R, et al. Management of chronic recurrent parotitis: current therapy. J Oral Maxillofac Surg 2004;62:1150–5.

14. Nichols RD. Surgical treatment of chronic suppurative parotitis. A critical review. Laryngoscope 1977; 87:2066–81.

15. Baurmash HD. Chronic recurrent parotitis: a closer look at its origin, diagnosis, and management. J Oral Maxillofac Surg 2004;62:1010–18.

16. Mandel L, Witek EL. Chronic parotitis. Diagnosis and treatment. J Am Dent Assoc 2001;132:1707–11.

17. Jungehulsing M, Fischbach R, Schroder U, et al. Magnetic resonance sialography. Otolaryngol Head Neck Surg 1999;121:488–94.

18. Galili D, Marmary Y. Spontaneous regeneration of the parotid salivary gland following juvenile recurrent parotitis. Oral Surg Oral Med Oral Pathol 1985;60:605–6.

19. Drage NA, Wilson RF, McGurk M. The genu of the submandibular duct—is the angle significant in salivary gland disease? Dentomaxillofac Radiol 2002; 31:15–8.
20. Yoshihara T, Kanada T, Yaku Y, et al. Chronic sialadenitis of the submandibular gland (so-called Kuttner tumor). Auris Nasus Larynx 1983;10:117–23.
21. Homes S, Gleeson MJ, Cawson RA. Mycobacterial disease of the parotid gland. Oral Surg Oral Med Oral Pathol Oral Radiol Endod 2000;90:292–8.
22. O'Connell JE, George MK, Speculand B, et al. Mycobacteria infection of the parotid gland: an unusual cause of parotid swelling. J Laryngol Otol 1993;107: 561–4.
23. Arrieta AJ, McCaffrey TV. Inflammatory disorders of the salivary glands. In: Cummings CW, editor. Cummings otolaryngology: head and neck surgery. 4th edition. Philadelphia: Elsevier Mosby; 2005. p. 1323–38.
24. Murray PR, Kobayashi GS, Pfaller KS. Paramyxoviruses. In: Medical microbiology. 2nd edition. St. Louis (MO): Mosby; 1994. p. 629–40.
25. deB Norman JE, Mitchell RD. Unusual conditions of the major and minor salivary glands. Int J Oral Maxillofac Surg 1998;27:157–72.

Indications, Techniques, and Complications of Major Salivary Gland Extirpation

Amy K. Hsu, MD, David I. Kutler, MD*

KEYWORDS

- Salivary gland • Parotid gland • Submandibular gland
- Surgery • Complications

The management of salivary gland diseases has evolved greatly with improvements in radiologic imaging and preoperative diagnostic techniques such as fine-needle aspiration biopsy (FNAB). Surgical management of the salivary gland is often indicated for a variety of inflammatory and neoplastic diseases. The major salivary glands are closely related to major neurovascular structures that require intraoperative management. Knowledge of these disease processes and anatomic relationships is essential to appropriate surgical management of the salivary glands. In this article we review major salivary gland anatomy, differential diagnosis, indications for surgical management, surgical technique for gland excision, and management of surgical complications. We conclude with a discussion of recent technological advances in salivary gland surgery.

ANATOMY

The salivary glands produce saliva in response to neural and humoral stimulation. The paired major salivary glands include the parotid glands, submandibular glands, and the sublingual glands. There are also approximately 500 to 1000 minor salivary glands interspersed throughout the mucosal surfaces of the lips, oral cavity, hard and soft palate, and pharynx.

Parotid Gland Anatomy

The parotid gland is the largest salivary gland and is located in the parotid compartment, a triangular space anterior and inferior to the auricle. Also contained in this space are the facial nerve (cranial nerve VII), numerous sensory and autonomic nerves, the external carotid artery and its branches, the retromandibular vein, and parotid lymphatics. The parotid is an irregular wedge-shaped gland that wraps around the posterior edge of the ramus of the mandible and extends posteriorly to the external auditory canal and mastoid tip. Approximately 80% of the gland overlies the masseter muscle anteriorly. The remaining 20% extends medially through the stylomandibular tunnel, which is bordered by the posterior edge of the mandibular ramus, the posterior belly of the digastric muscle, the upper portion of the sternocleidomastoid muscle, and the stylomandibular ligament.[1] The stylomandibular ligament extends from the styloid process to the mandible and also separates the parotid gland from the submandibular gland. The parotid fascia incompletely covers the gland and is a continuation of the superficial layer of the deep cervical fascia. The facial nerve traverses through the parotid gland and artificially divides it into superficial and deep lobes. The superficial or lateral lobe is larger and consists of the parotid tissue lateral to the facial nerve. The deep lobe lies medial to the facial nerve and anterior to the styloid process in the

Department of Otorhinolaryngology, Head and Neck Surgery, New York Presbyterian Hospital, Weill Medical College of Cornell University, 1305 York Avenue, 5th Floor, New York, NY 10021, USA
* Corresponding author.
E-mail address: dik2002@med.cornell.edu (D.I. Kutler).

Oral Maxillofacial Surg Clin N Am 21 (2009) 313–321
doi:10.1016/j.coms.2009.04.001
1042-3699/09/$ – see front matter © 2009 Elsevier Inc. All rights reserved.

prestyloid portion of the parapharyngeal space. In addition to the deep lobe of the parotid gland, the prestyloid portion of the parapharyngeal space contains fat and lymphatics. The poststyloid portion contains the internal carotid artery, internal jugular vein, cranial nerves IX to XII, and the cervical sympathetic chain.

The facial nerve is intimately associated with the parotid gland, and understanding its anatomy is critical to successful parotid surgery. The facial nerve exits the skull base at the stylomastoid foramen. It gives off branches to the stylohyoid, postauricular, and posterior belly of the digastric muscles before turning anterolaterally to enter the parotid gland. At the pes anserinus, the facial

nerve splits into two major divisions, the zygomaticotemporal (upper) and cervicofacial (lower). With some variation, these divisions give rise to the five terminal branches: zygomatic, temporal, buccal, marginal mandibular, and cervical. Davis[2] described six different facial nerve branching patterns with no predominant pattern (**Fig. 1**). In all types, the temporal and zygomatic branches arise from the upper division, and the cervical and marginal mandibular branches arise from the lower division. The major variations are in the origin of the buccal branch and the degree of cross innervation between adjacent terminal branches. In type I, the buccal branch originates from the upper division, and the five terminal branches do

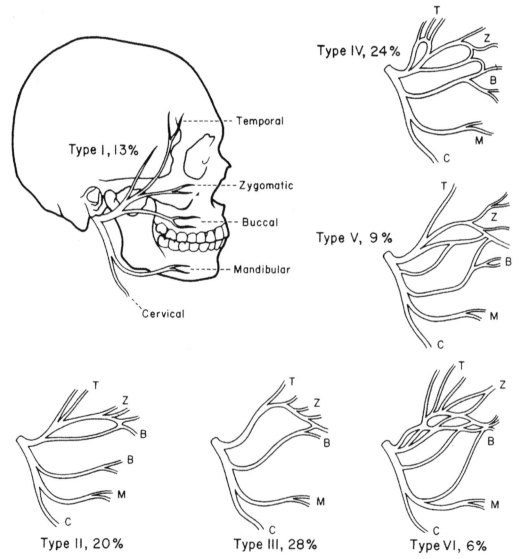

Fig. 1. Anatomic variations in branching patterns of the facial nerve. (*Adapted from* Davis RA, Anson BJ, Budinger JM, et al. Surgical anatomy of the facial nerve and parotid gland based upon a study of 350 cervicofacial halves. Surg Gynecol Obstet (now J Am Coll Surg) 1956;102:405; with permission.)

not cross innervate. In type II, buccal branches originate from both the upper and lower divisions, and there is cross innervation between buccal and zygomatic branches in the upper division. In types III–VI, the buccal branches arise primarily from the lower division and traverse superiorly to join the upper division terminal fibers. These types have an increasing amount of branching and cross innervation among the upper division branches, with type VI having the most branches.[2] In general, the buccal and zygomatic branches have the greatest amount of cross innervation.

The parotid duct or Stensen's duct courses anteriorly along a path parallel to the zygomatic arch approximately 1 to 1.5 cm below the inferior border of the arch. It travels superficial to the masseter muscle and then turns medially at a right angle to pierce the buccinator muscle. The parotid duct lies midway between the zygomatic arch and the oral commissure along a line drawn between the philtrum of the upper lip and the tragus. The duct empties into the oral cavity at the parotid papilla, a small elevation of tissue across from the second maxillary molar. Accessory parotid glands are found in approximately 20% of patients. They typically overlie the masseter muscle; their ductal systems are separate and may or may not be contiguous with Stensen's duct. Benign or malignant neoplasms can infrequently involve the accessory parotid glands and should be considered when a mass is very anteriorly located in the parotid region.

The secretory function of the gland is controlled via parasympathetic efferents from the inferior salivatory nucleus via the glossopharyngeal nerve and sympathetic nerves from the superior cervical ganglion. The arterial supply is from branches off the external carotid artery, primarily the transverse facial artery from the superficial temporal artery. Venous drainage is primarily via the retromandibular vein, which drains to both the external and internal jugular veins. The parotid gland has a rich lymphatic supply. Paraparotid lymph nodes are located superficial to the capsule and drain the temporal region, scalp, and auricle. Intraparotid lymph nodes are embedded in the parenchyma and receive drainage from the ear, soft palate, and posterior nasopharynx. The parotid and intraparotid lymph nodes drain into the superficial and deep cervical lymph node chains.

Submandibular Gland Anatomy

The submandibular gland occupies the submandibular triangle, the space bordered by the inferior border of the mandible and the anterior and posterior bellies of the digastric muscle. The gland is C-shaped and wraps around the mylohyoid muscle, which divides it into superficial and deep lobes. The deep component comprises the majority of the gland. The submandibular gland is invested by a capsule that is contiguous with the superficial layer of the deep cervical fascia, which also contains the marginal mandibular branch of the facial nerve. The marginal mandibular nerve originates from the lower division of the facial nerve. It courses inferiorly over the angle of the mandible and then loops to course anterosuperiorly. The marginal mandibular nerve provides motor innervation to the depressor muscles of the lip, and injury results in a lower facial asymmetry. The facial artery arises from the external carotid artery and runs deep to the digastric muscle and submandibular gland and then courses superiorly over the mandible toward the face. The submandibular gland is supplied by the submental branch of the facial artery. The facial vein travels near the facial artery on the lateral surface of the gland. The marginal mandibular nerve is superficial to the facial artery and vein.

The submandibular ducts, or Wharton's ducts, emanate from deep within the gland and exit on its medial surface between the mylohyoid and hyoglossus muscles. The submandibular ducts empty into the floor of the mouth on either side of the frenulum and are closely associated with both the hypoglossal and lingual nerves. The hypoglossal nerve parallels the duct and runs deep in the submandibular space, deep to the digastric muscle and to the gland itself. The lingual nerve courses laterally to the duct and then loops inferiorly and passes medial to the duct.

Sympathetic innervation to the submandibular gland arises from the superior cervical ganglion. Parasympathetic innervation is from the lingual nerve via the submandibular ganglion. Lymphatic drainage is to the deep cervical, jugular, and perivascular lymph nodes near the facial artery.

Histopathology of the Secretory Unit

The basic subunit of the salivary gland is the secretory unit, which consists of an acinus, a secretory duct, and a collecting duct. The acinus is comprised of pyramidal-shaped secretory cells framing a central lumen that drains into the intercalated duct followed by the striated duct. The acini in the parotid are serous and produce watery saliva, whereas the submandibular gland contains mixed (serous and mucous) acini that produce semiviscous saliva. The acini and intercalated ducts are surrounded by elongated nonsecretory cells called myoepithelial cells that may play a contractile role in secreting saliva.[3] The intercalated and striated ducts are intralobular ducts that drain into larger extralobular collecting ducts, or excretory ducts. Although the sublingual and minor salivary glands secrete saliva via many collecting ducts, the parotid and submandibular glands have several interlobular ducts that secrete via a single large collecting duct.

DIFFERENTIAL DIAGNOSIS OF THE SALIVARY GLANDS

The spectrum of salivary pathology includes acute and chronic inflammatory, infectious, neoplastic, and obstructive processes. These disorders have a wide range of clinical presentations but frequently manifest as either an isolated mass or a diffusely enlarged gland. Both medical and surgical therapies play a role in the management of salivary gland disorders. A summary of the differential diagnosis for salivary gland disease can be found in **Table 1**. The following section is not all inclusive and focuses on the most frequently encountered salivary gland diseases.

Acute Inflammatory Disorders

An acute painful swelling of the salivary gland usually suggests an inflammatory process most

Table 1
Differential diagnosis of salivary gland diseases

Salivary Gland Diseases	Differential Diagnosis
Inflammatory Disorders	
Bacterial Sialadenitis	Acute Chronic Paramyxovirus (mumps)
Viral Infection	HIV Tuberculosis Atypical mycobacterial infection
Granulomatous	Toxoplasmosis Cat scratch disease Actinomycosis Sarcoidosis
Autoimmune	Sjögren's
Obstructive Disorders	Sialolithiasis Ductal stenosis Ductal stricture Mucus plug Congenital dilation
Cystic Lesions	Lymphoepithelial cyst Branchial cleft cyst Mucocele Mucus retention cyst
Other Tumor-Like	Sialadenosis Necrotizing sialometaplasia Kuttner tumor
Benign Neoplasms	Pleomorphic adenoma Warthin's tumor (papillary cystadenoma lymphomatosum) Monomorphic adenoma Oncocytoma Hemangioma
Malignant Neoplasms	Mucoepidermoid carcinoma Adenoid cystic carcinoma Acinic cell carcinoma Malignant mixed tumor Adenocarcinoma Epithelial-myoepithelial carcinoma Squamous cell carcinoma Lymphoma Melanoma

often bacterial or viral in origin. Bacterial infection of the salivary gland, or bacterial sialadenitis, can occur as a result of salivary stasis and retrograde infiltration of bacteria into the gland. The infection usually presents with a swollen, erythematous, and tender gland. Purulence may be expressed from the ductal orifice during palpation of the gland. Initial management is medical and consists of antibiotics, hydration, warm compresses, sialogogues, gland massage, and oral irrigations. Despite the above therapies, the infection may progress to an abscess requiring surgical incision and drainage. The treatment for viral infection is primarily supportive care. Management of acute sialadenitis should also address predisposing medical conditions, such as dehydration, advanced age, prior radiation, and immunocompromise.

Chronic Inflammatory Disorders

Chronic sialadenitis is characterized by recurrent painful swelling of the salivary gland, usually the parotid. This condition usually occurs as a result of salivary duct obstruction and salivary stasis. Obstruction can occur as a result of sialolithiasis, ductal stricture, extrinsic tumor compression, stenosis from adjacent scar tissue, or congenital ductal dilation. Repeated episodes of infection and inflammation can lead to ductal ectasia and acinar destruction. Patients typically have episodes of tender gland enlargement interspersed with asymptomatic periods of weeks to months. Treatment is similar to that of acute sialadenitis and involves hydration, analgesics, and antibiotics. Because of the degree of scarring and parenchymal damage that occurs from chronic inflammation, surgical excision in chronic sialadenitis carries an increased risk of complications such as bleeding or facial nerve injury. Hence, gland excision should be considered only in patients with significant pain and symptoms refractory to conservative therapy.

Salivary gland enlargement can also be caused by autoimmune disorders such as Sjögren's disease or by granulomatous diseases, including tuberculosis, nontuberculous mycobacterial infection, sarcoidosis, actinomycosis, and cat scratch disease. Treatment is usually nonsurgical and is directed toward the underlying cause.

Excision of the salivary gland may be indicated for diagnosis or treatment in some conditions, especially those refractory to medical therapy. However, surgery plays a limited role in the management of most chronic inflammatory processes of the salivary gland.

OPERATIVE TECHNIQUES
Superficial Parotidectomy

Superficial parotidectomy is indicated for most benign and malignant tumors in the superficial lobe, for chronic sialadenitis, and as part of a lymphadenectomy for skin cancer of the scalp. Parotid masses should not be enucleated because of risk of tumor recurrence and the increased risk to the facial nerve during revision surgery. Tumors that extend into the deep lobe may require total parotidectomy including both the superficial and deep lobes.[1]

The modified Blair incision for superficial parotidectomy begins in a natural crease just anterior to the helix, extends underneath the earlobe and superiorly over the mastoid, and then curves inferiorly over the anterior border of the sternocleidomastoid muscle. The incision continues below the angle of the mandible at a distance safe from the marginal mandibular nerve (two finger breadths). Placing the incision posterior rather than anterior to the tragus may improve the cosmetic result. Dissection is carried sharply to the depth of the parotid fascia in the preauricular region and through the platysma muscle in the cervical region. Anterior and posterior flaps are raised along this plane, exposing the gland anteriorly and the anterior border of the sternocleidomastoid muscle posteriorly. Care should be taken to not "button-hole" the skin flap by raising an excessively thin flap. The flaps are then sutured in place or retracted away from the surgical field.

Using sharp dissection, the tail of the parotid gland is then separated from the sternocleidomastoid muscle, the cartilaginous external auditory canal, and the posterior digastric and stylohyoid muscles. The greater auricular nerve is encountered during mobilization of the lateral lobe. Its anterior division must usually be sacrificed to mobilize the gland adequately. If possible, the posterior division of the greater auricular nerve should be preserved to maintain sensation to the earlobe.[4] The tragal pointer and tympanomastoid suture line are also exposed during this dissection.

Attention is then focused on the critical task of localizing the facial nerve. Several surgical landmarks aid in the identification of the seventh nerve.

Tragal pointer
The main trunk of the facial nerve is located 1 cm anteroinferior and 1 cm deep to the tip of the tragal cartilage.

Digastric ridge
The main trunk is just superior to the attachment of the posterior belly of the digastric muscle to the

digastric groove. This landmark also marks the approximate depth of the facial nerve.

Stylomastoid foramen

The base of the styloid process is 5 to 8 mm deep to the tympanomastoid suture line. The facial nerve can be identified as it exits the stylomastoid foramen and passes over the posterolateral aspect of the styloid process.

Tympanomastoid suture line

The nerve lies 6 to 8 mm deep to the inferior end of the tympanomastoid suture line.

Mastoid

For revision cases, extensive tumors or, as a last resort, a mastoidectomy can be performed to locate the vertical segment of the facial nerve, which can then be followed as it exits the mastoid.

The facial nerve may also be identified in a retrograde fashion by tracing a terminal branch proximally. Several key relationships are helpful in identification of one or more terminal branches. The cervical branch of the facial nerve is just lateral to the posterior division of the retromandibular vein. The marginal mandibular nerve courses along the inferior border of the parotid gland and passes superficial to the retromandibular vein. The buccal branch travels with the parotid duct and usually lies just superior to the duct. The temporal branch crosses the zygomatic arch midway between the tragus and lateral canthus, anterior to the superficial temporal artery and vein.[5]

After the main trunk of the facial nerve is localized, the pes anserinus is exposed and followed as it branches into the zygomaticotemporal and cervicofacial divisions. Each terminal nerve branch should be traced meticulously in a contiguous fashion, as skipping sections of nerve increases the likelihood of nerve injury. Every attempt should be made to spare the facial nerve and its terminal branches. However, resection of the nerve may be indicated for direct tumor involvement or encasement of the nerve. The decision to preserve or sacrifice the nerve must frequently be made intraoperatively. The use of intraoperative facial nerve monitoring, an operating microscope, or a nerve stimulator may aid in the intraoperative localization and preservation of nerve branches. Although the use of intraoperative monitoring may provide useful feedback intraoperatively, its routine use is controversial given increased cost and operating time without clear improvement in outcomes.[6–8]

The parotid gland is then grasped and retracted with Allis clamps, while a fine curved clamp is used to carefully dissect each branch of the facial nerve from the gland parenchyma. The superficial lobe is separated from the deep lobe in a similar fashion. The superior margin of the gland is then dissected free, taking care to avoid injury to the zygomatic and temporal branches. Near the terminal fibers of the buccal branch, Stensen's duct is identified and ligated. After removal of the gland, hemostasis is achieved using a bipolar cautery. A small drain, usually a Jackson-Pratt, is placed in the cervical portion of the wound. The incision is closed using nylon sutures in the preauricular area and a standard layered closure in the neck. A pressure dressing is sometimes placed to prevent hematoma and seroma formation.

Early complications

The main trunk of the facial nerve or any of its extratemporal branches can be injured intraoperatively during a parotidectomy. The nerve may be stretched or crushed, resulting in a temporary facial weakness, or it may be transected, resulting in permanent facial paralysis. If the nerve is transected or sacrificed intraoperatively it should be repaired immediately with primary neurorrhaphy or cable grafting if the nerve branches are under tension. The greater auricular nerve and sural nerve are commonly used for cable grafting in this circumstance. Postoperative weakness and delayed paralysis usually resolve and can be managed conservatively with observation, steroids, and electrodiagnostic studies. Complete postoperative paralysis after intraoperative confirmation of nerve preservation may warrant reexploration in select cases.

Greater auricular nerve paresthesia is expected if the nerve is transected intraoperatively. Patients should be counseled preoperatively to expect numbness over the auricle. Hematoma and seroma formation are infrequent complications. Their incidence can be minimized by careful hemostasis intraoperatively and suction drain placement before closure; a pressure dressing may also be placed. Treatment for hematoma is wound exploration, evacuation, and hemostasis with bipolar cautery to avoid thermal injury to the facial nerve. Seromas place the patient at increased risk for wound infection and should be treated with repeated needle aspiration until the collection resolves. Salivary fistula is a less common complication that is treated with anticholinergic medications and a pressure dressing.[9]

Late complications

Tumor recurrence may occur in benign or malignant lesions, particularly if an enucleation or incomplete lobectomy is performed. Recurrence is problematic as significant fibrosis may be present around the facial nerve. If revision surgery is indicated, facial nerve monitoring should be considered.

Gustatory sweating, also known as Frey's syndrome, presents as redness and perspiration over the cheek and parotid region in anticipation of eating. This complication may develop several years after parotidectomy and occurs when severed parasympathetic nerves to the parotid gland regenerate in an aberrant fashion and innervate sweat glands in the dermis. Some surgeons advocate thicker skin flaps, placement of acellular dermis (AlloDerm), fat grafting, or interpostion flaps to prevent this complication. Nonsurgical therapies for Frey's syndrome include botulinum toxin A injections, anticholinergic creams, and topical antiperspirants. If medical therapies fail, the aforementioned surgical techniques can also be performed as a second procedure to alleviate symptoms. Additionally, middle ear exploration and tympanic neurectomy have been attempted with some success.[10]

Patients will have some degree of cosmetic deformity after parotid surgery. Usually after superficial parotidectomy, the degree of depression is not severe. For large cosmetic defects, such as after total parotidectomy, locoregional flaps may be used to provide tissue bulk. However, these flaps may make detection of recurrent lesions difficult on physical examination.

Submandibular Gland Resection

Submandibular gland removal is indicated for sialolithiasis, refractory chronic sialadenitis, and benign and malignant neoplasms. A horizontal skin incision is made in a natural skin crease that is at least two finger breadths (4 cm) below the inferior border of the mandible to avoid injury to the marginal mandibular nerve. The incision extends from the middle of the ipsilateral digastric tendon to the anterior border of the sternocleidomastoid muscle. The dissection is then carried through the platysma muscle to the level of the superficial layer of the deep cervical fascia. Upper and lower flaps are raised in the plane between the platysma and the superficial layer of the deep cervical fascia. The marginal nerve lies just deep to the cervical fascia and superficial to the facial artery and facial vein. A safe way to preserve the marginal nerve is to ligate the facial vein and incise the submandibular gland fascia at the inferior border of the gland. These tissues can then be lifted from the gland along with the marginal nerve. The marginal nerve usually lies superior to the

inferior border of the gland. However, during its course it may drape inferior to the vessels and may be encountered unexpectedly before the facial vein is identified. An even safer approach is to identify the nerve while raising the superior flap, before the ligation of the facial vein. The nerve can thus be kept in view at all times, decreasing the risk of transection or stretch injury.

The excision of the gland is begun at the lower border of the gland. At this juncture, the hypoglossal nerve should be identified adjacent to the intermediate tendon of the digastric muscle. The dissection is then carried superiorly in the plane between the digastric muscle and the submandibular gland. The facial artery is encountered on the posterior aspect of the gland as it passes deep to the posterior belly of the digastric and enters the submandibular gland. The facial artery is then ligated, taking care to preserve the hypoglossal nerve. By gentle anterior retraction of the mylohyoid muscle, the deep lobe of the submandibular gland is exposed.[1] The lingual nerve and efferent fibers of the chorda tympani can be identified deep to the mylohyoid muscle along with the submandibular ganglion. Just medial to the lingual nerve is Wharton's duct. The submandibular duct, lingual nerve, and hypoglossal nerve should be identified before excision of the gland. The submandibular gland is easily removed after ligation of its pedicle and Wharton's duct. The preserved lingual nerve is left in place deep to the mylohyoid muscle. If malignancy is suspected, a submandibular lymph node dissection should be performed, including removal of perivascular nodes near the facial artery. High grade malignancies or malignancies with lymph node metastases may also require a complete neck dissection to remove metastatic disease. A small suction drain can be placed prior to closing the platysma muscle. A layered closure should be performed, including approximation of the platysma muscle, deep dermal sutures, and skin closure.

Complications

Complications of submandibular gland excision include bleeding, infection, seroma formation, and damage to the marginal mandibular nerve. Weakness of depressor muscles of the lower lip is the most common complication of a submandibular gland excision. Temporary weakness may occur from transection of the platysma muscle, which aids in depression of the lip with its insertion into the depressor labi inferioris and depressor anguli oris.[11] Return of platysma function usually occurs if the muscle is well approximated during wound closure. Transient weakness can also occur from stretch injury to the marginal nerve during surgery. However, if the marginal mandibular nerve is transected, loss of lower lip depressor function is permanent. If there is no return in function after 9 to 12 months, a lip suspension procedure can be performed to aid in oral competence and improve cosmetic appearance. The lingual and hypoglossal nerves can also be injured during submandibular gland surgery.

The management of postoperative hematoma is wound exploration, clot evacuation, and hemostasis with bipolar cautery to avoid thermal injury to the marginal mandibular nerve. Seroma formation after submandibular gland excision is usually treated with compression and serial needle aspirations of the serous fluid.

Long-term considerations include recurrence of sialadenitis and cosmetic deformity. Patients undergoing surgery for sialolithiasis may have recurrence of stones in the residual Wharton's duct.[12] Additionally, patients may note a depression at the site of the gland excision after postoperative swelling resolves. Usually this defect does not pose a significant cosmetic problem.

FUTURE DIRECTIONS

The growing trend toward minimally invasive surgical procedures along with recent technological advances has greatly increased the number of conservative therapeutic options for the management of benign obstructive processes of the salivary glands. Many investigators have reported successful treatment of ductal strictures and sialoliths in both the submandibular and parotid glands using combinations of sialendoscopy, fluoroscopic basket retrieval, extracorporeal shock wave lithotripsy, and laser intracorporeal lithotripsy.[13-15] In particular, sialendoscopy has increased in popularity with the development of high-resolution salivary endoscopes and accompanying retrieval instruments. With the use of grasping forceps, wire baskets, balloons, and stents, obstructive lesions can be treated with success rates as high as 80% to 90%.[16] Some authors have reported a decrease in the rate of sialadenectomy to less than 5% with the use of these approaches.[13,17]

Intraoral resection of the submandibular gland has also been described as an alternative to the transcervical approach.[18] Benefits include lack of scar and decreased risk to the marginal mandibular nerve. Hong reported successful removal of the submandibular gland in 77 patients with benign disorders. However, temporary lingual sensory paresis and limitation of tongue movement occurred in 74% and 70% of patients, respectively.[19]

Minimally invasive techniques have also been employed for patients who require gland excision. Chen published a small series of patients who successfully underwent endoscope-assisted excision of the submandibular gland for benign lesions via a midline incision at the level of the hyoid.[20] Some surgeons have also performed endoscope-assisted parotidectomy for benign parotid lesions via a postauricular skin incision. Preliminary results show a low rate of facial nerve injury in two limited series of patients.[21,22]

Many of these new technologies are expensive, require increased operating time, and must overcome a learning curve on the part of the surgeon operators. As their use increases, it remains to be determined whether these techniques will provide equivalent outcomes and complication rates.

SUMMARY

Surgical techniques for salivary gland surgery will continue to evolve as new technologies develop. A thorough understanding of the disease processes and anatomy will remain of paramount importance in the successful surgical management of salivary gland disease.

REFERENCES

1. Futran ND, Parvathaneni U, Martins RG, et al. Malignant salivary gland tumors. Part A: general principles and management. In: Harrison LB, Sessions RB, Hong WK, editors. Head and neck cancer: a multidisciplinary approach. 3rd edition. Philadelphia: Lippincott Williams & Wilkins; 2009. p. 589–610.
2. Davis RA, Anson BJ, Budinger JM, et al. Surgical anatomy of the facial nerve and parotid gland based upon a study of 350 cervicofacial halves. Surg Gynecol Obstet 1956;102(4):385–412.
3. Elluru RG, Kumar M, et al. Physiology of the salivary glands. In: Cummings CW, Haughey BH, Thomas JR, et al, editors. Cummings otolaryngology: head and neck surgery, 4th edition 2. Philadelphia: Mosby Inc.; 2005. p. 1293–312.
4. Lore J, Medina J. The parotid salivary gland and management of malignant salivary gland neoplasia. In: Lore J, Medina J, editors. An atlas of head and neck surgery. 4th edition. Philadelphia: WB Saunders; 2004. p. 861–91.
5. Sinha UK, Ng M. Surgery of the salivary glands. Otolaryngol Clin North Am 1999;32(5):887–906.
6. Dulguerov P, Marchal F, Lehmann W. Postparotidectomy facial nerve paralysis: possible etiologic factors and results with routine facial nerve monitoring. Laryngoscope 1999;109(5):754–62.

7. Meier JD, Wenig BL, Manders EC, et al. Continuous intraoperative facial nerve monitoring in predicting postoperative injury during parotidectomy. Laryngoscope 2006;116(9):1569–72.

8. Terrell JE, Kileny PR, Yian C, et al. Clinical outcome of continuous facial nerve monitoring during primary parotidectomy. Arch Otolaryngol Head Neck Surg 1997;123(10):1081–7.

9. Cavanaugh K, Park A. Postparotidectomy fistula: a different treatment for an old problem. Int J Pediatr Otorhinolaryngol 1999;47(3):265–8.

10. Simental A, Carrau RL, et al. Malignant neoplasms of the salivary glands. In: Cummings CW, Haughey BH, Thomas JR, et al, editors. Cummings otolaryngology: head and neck surgery 4th edition 2. Philadelphia: Mosby Inc.; 2005. p. 1378–405.

11. Lore J, Medina J. The neck. In: Lore J, Medina J, editors. An atlas of head and neck surgery. 4th edition. Philadelphia: Saunders; 2004. p. 780–860.

12. Williams MF. Sialolithiasis. Otolaryngol Clin North Am 1999;32(5):819–34.

13. Capaccio P, Torretta S, Ottavian F, et al. Modern management of obstructive salivary diseases. Acta Otorhinolaryngol Ital 2007;27(4):161–72.

14. Drage NA, Brown JE, Escudier MP, et al. Interventional radiology in the removal of salivary calculi. Radiology 2000;214(1):139–42.

15. McGurk M, Escudier MP, Brown E. Modern management of obstructive salivary gland disease. Ann R Australas Coll Dent Surg 2004; 17:45–50.

16. Nahlieli O, Nakar LH, Nazarian Y, et al. Sialoendoscopy: a new approach to salivary gland obstructive pathology. J Am Dent Assoc 2006;137(10): 1394–400.

17. Lari N, Chossegros C, Thiery G, et al. [Sialendoscopy of the salivary glands]. Rev Stomatol Chir Maxillofac 2008;109(3):167–71 [in French].

18. Hong KH, Kim YK. Intraoral removal of the submandibular gland: a new surgical approach. Otolaryngol Head Neck Surg 2000;122(6): 798–802.

19. Hong KH, Yang YS. Surgical results of the intraoral removal of the submandibular gland. Otolaryngol Head Neck Surg 2008;139(4):530–4.

20. Chen MK, Su CC, Tsai YL, et al. Minimally invasive endoscopic resection of the submandibular gland: a new approach. Head Neck 2006;28(11):1014–7.

21. Chen MK, Chang CC. Minimally invasive endoscope-assisted parotidectomy: a new approach. Laryngoscope 2007;117(11):1934–7.

22. Gao L, Shao Y, Xie L, et al. Endoscope-assisted parotidectomy for benign tumors via a short hidden auricular incision. Zhonghua Zheng Xing Wai Ke Za Zhi 2004;20(4):290–3.

Sialoendoscopy and Salivary Gland Sparing Surgery

Michael D. Turner, DDS, MD, FACS

KEYWORDS

- Sialoendoscopy • Salivary gland • Sialoadenitis
- Parotitis • Endoscopy • Minimally invasive surgery

Obstructive disease and chronic infections often are managed by extirpative gland surgery. Even in cases when surgery is limited to distal structures of the gland, loss of function and glandular integrity are inevitable. With the advent of new technology and better understanding of salivary physiology, minimally invasive surgical techniques provide the opportunity, not only for safer and less invasive surgery in alternative care settings, but also the prospect for gland sparing and restoration of normal function. This article describes techniques for managing acute and chronic salivary gland infections using sialoendoscopy.

HISTORY

Independently, Krönensberg and Gundlach published the first use of sialoendoscopy for ablation of a salivary duct stone in conjunction with endoscopic visualization.[1–3] Katz, a radiologist, published a technique for the visualization of sialoliths using a 0.8 mm flexible endoscope. Krönensberg introduced a flexible endoscope in combination with an intracorporeal lithotripter in 1993.[4] The technique of using a rigid endoscope was introduced concurrently in 1994 by Arzoz, who employed a 2.1 mm rigid miniurethroscope with a working channel of 1 mm, and Nahlieli, who used a 2.7 mm arthroscope.[5,6] Following cadaveric studies by Zenk, Marchal duplicated the sialoendoscopic techniques using a 2 mm endoscope, but then decreased the size of the endoscope.[7] Zenk's studies revealed that the average diameter of the Stensen's duct ranged from 0.5 to 1.4 mm, with a minimum of 0.1 mm and a maximum of 2.3 mm, depending on the location. They concluded that endoscopes should not exceed the diameter of 1.2 mm.[8]

TECHNOLOGY: SIALOENDOSCOPES

The sialoendoscope is a small endoscope that can be introduced intraorally into the salivary gland using a major salivary gland duct. There are two mandatory components to a sialoendoscope, the optical fibers and an irrigation port. The optical fibers typically are encased in a semirigid material. They come as a self-contained unit with irrigation or working port(s), or they can be introduced into a sheath that contains irrigation or working ports (**Fig. 1**). The diameter of the total unit is the limiting factor. Generally, it is difficult to introduce a sialoendoscope without an incision into the duct when the diameter of the endoscope is 1.3 mm or greater. At the diameter of 1.2 mm, a stent must be introduced to prevent scarring caused by adhesion formation within the distal portion of the salivary duct (**Fig. 2**).

INDICATIONS FOR SIALOENDOSCOPY

Sialoendoscopy has been proven to be most effective for correcting salivary gland obstructions. There are generally four different types of salivary ductal obstructions: mucous plugs, foreign bodies, sialolithiasis, and strictures/adhesions.

Mucous Plugs

Mucous plugs present with general symptoms of salivary obstruction. The gland expands following salivary stimulation and lack of salivary flow from the glandular duct, with no exudate being

Department of Oral and Maxillofacial Surgery, New York University College of Dentistry, 345 East 24th Street, New York, NY 10010, USA
E-mail address: mdt4@nyu.edu

Oral Maxillofacial Surg Clin N Am 21 (2009) 323–329
doi:10.1016/j.coms.2009.05.003

oralmaxsurgery.theclinics.com

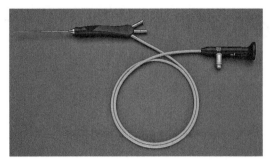

Fig.1. Image of a Karl Storz sialoendoscope. (*Courtesy of* KARL STORZ Endoscopy-America, Inc., El Segundo, CA; with permission.)

expressed. Patients most likely will not have a history of prior obstruction. It most commonly occurs in the submandibular gland, secondary to the high mucous content of its saliva. Resolution generally is obtained without intervention and occurs spontaneously and quickly. If obstruction does not resolve within 2 hours, conservative intervention should be considered. Rehydration therapy is typically effective by increasing the serous content of the submandibular saliva, and thus, the mucous plug begins to dissolve from contact with the now less viscous saliva. Rehydration can be achieved by oral ingestion of 2 L of nonalcoholic fluid, or by intravenous infusion of lactated ringers, or other appropriate solutions.

If resolution does not occur following rehydration, simple interventions may be attempted. A small lacrimal probe can be introduced into the gland, dislodging the plug. If navigation of the duct is difficult, a small (22 or 24 gauge) intravenous catheter (sans needle) can be placed into the gland, and then 1 mL of fluid (eg, sterile saline) can be infused into the gland, loosening the

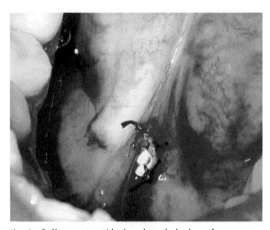

Fig. 2. Salivary stent/drain placed during the surgery to prevent adhesion formation.

mucous plug. If conservative management is not successful, sialoendoscopy is indicated. The smallest diameter (less than 1.0 mm) sialoendoscope should be used. The mucous plug is dislodged by irrigation fluid, the endoscope, microinstruments, or a combination of all three.

Foreign Bodies

There are several case reports of various foreign bodies that have been found within the submandibular duct or gland. Many of these cases are found in children who have placed an object into their mouths. Objects that have been identified are: grass, hay, wood, food debris, popcorn kernels, and one reported case of a large fishbone within the submandibular duct. These bodies, if not dislodged by salivary flow, should be removed because of their ability to occlude the duct and to act as a nidus of infection. Foreign bodies are difficult to visualize using radiographic and ultrasound techniques. They normally are identified when they are expelled from the duct naturally, or when they are removed using a sialoendoscopic technique. Patients should be placed on antibiotics because of the contamination of the sterile salivary gland system.

Sialolithiasis

Sialolithiasis is the most common cause of obstruction in the major salivary glands. A recent study of 877 cases of proven obstruction revealed that 73.2% were caused by salivary stones, while 22.6% were caused by salivary duct stricture formation without evidence of stones.[9] Like mucous plugs, salivary stones are located most frequently in the submandibular glands (80% to 90%), with most of the remainder in the parotid glands. A very small percentage of calculi is found in the sublingual glands, but this is not clinically significant as an independent disease process. Management is discussed further in the technique section of this article.

Strictures

Salivary duct stenosis is a narrowing of the duct lumen sufficient to cause a decrease or complete cessation of salivary flow. These strictures may present as singular or multiple entities. There are two types of isolated strictures, congenital and traumatic. A very common congenital stricture in the parotid gland is the area where the parotid duct crosses through the buccinator muscle. Just from the compression of the buccinator muscle, a narrowing of the canal can occur. This is generally not clinically significant because of the high pressure of salivary expression from the effect on the masseteric.

Sling's compression on the parotid gland. Another region of narrowing is the location of the confluence of the submandibular duct and the lingual nerve. As the lingual nerve passes superior over the duct, a small compression of the duct can be visualized using sialoendoscopy. This is the anatomic explanation for lingual nerve paresthesia as discussed in the complications section. Isolated traumatic strictures can be iatrogenic or from dislodgement of fibrosed sialoliths or other foreign bodies. This dislodgement causes exposure of the ductal epithelium causing adhesion formation and narrowing or complete obstruction of the duct. Iatrogenic trauma from lacrimal probes or other inserted devices also can create adhesions. Most strictures (75.3%) are found in the parotid glands, with a higher predilection in females.[9]

Multiple diffuse strictures are seen from chronic infections or from underlying disease process. Chronic salivary gland infections increase the amount of inflammation and epithelium damage, leading to multiple strictures within the primary, secondary, and tertiary ductal systems. This also leads to the technical difficulty of introducing the sialoendoscopes into the gland. Careful visualization and dilation are necessary to prevent perforation and false passage of the endoscope.

TECHNIQUE

Before the introduction of the scope into the ductal system, the opening must be dilated. Lacrimal probes and dilators are needed to accomplish this aspect. Lacrimal probes are placed into the duct, starting at size 4–0, sequentially increasing in size to 8. This portion of the procedure is extremely important. If the probes are placed with excessive pressure, perforation of the duct into the surrounding tissues may occur. Once this occurs, it can be difficult to reintroduce the probes along the correct pathway, and extravasation of fluid into surrounding tissues is likely. Balloon dilation also can be performed within the distal portion of the duct using either salivary duct balloon dilators (sialotechnology), or size 3 or 4 Fogarty catheters (**Fig. 3**). Following successful dilation, the sialoendoscope is introduced into the gland opening; irrigation (normal saline or lactated ringers) is provided through one of the ports under pressure. This expands the duct and ductules away from the optical portion of the endoscope, allowing visualization of the duct and glandular tissues (**Fig. 4**). The initial portion of the surgery is the most productive and visible portion.

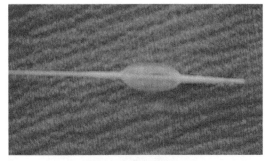

Fig. 3. Balloon dilator for the expansion of the duct, lysis of adhesion, and dilation of strictures.

If there has been sufficient extravasation of fluid into the surrounding areas, the ducts are constricted by the surrounding engorged salivary tissue, and visualization becomes impaired.

The types of surgery most conducive to pure endoscopic surgeries are: diagnostic sialoendoscopy, sialolithectomy, sialoendoscopic biopsy, and lysis of adhesions. Diagnostic sialoendoscopy generally is performed using a sialoendoscope with a diameter smaller than 1 mm. It does not have a working port, and it is used to evaluate the ductal system for pathology, or to evaluate the healing of the surgical site postoperatively. Sialolithectomy usually can be performed on sialolith, or sialolith fragments when their diameter is 7 mm or smaller (**Fig. 5**). When indicated, biopsy of the gland and the duct can be performed with biopsy forceps that can be introduced through the endoscope to the tissue in question. Caution should be observed. Although never documented

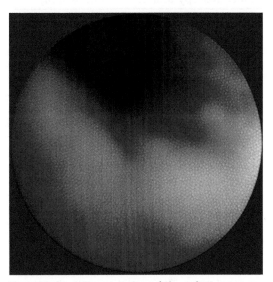

Fig. 4. Hydrostatic expansion of the soft tissues away from optic portion of the sialoendoscope.

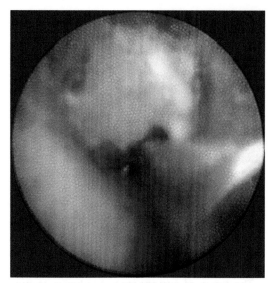

Fig. 5. Dissection of a sialolith away from the ductal tissues.

in this technique, mechanical seeding of abdominal tumors has occurred along the laparoscopic pathway when a laparoscopic resection of tumors has been attempted.[10] The final technique in which a pure sialoendoscopic technique can be used is in the lysis of adhesions and the dilation of strictures in the ductal system. Utilizing balloon dilators, dissection forceps, and the hydrostatic pressure of the irrigation canal, this surgery has been successful, particularly in case of juvenile recurrent parotitis.[11]

Sialoendoscopy-assisted Sialolithectomy

When a sialolith is too large to remove with just the sialoendoscope and the appropriate accessories, a sialoendoscopic-assisted sialolithectomy can be performed. The technique is used for removing a stone in conjunction with an intraoral or extraoral technique. In both procedures, the stone can be located by performing a diagnostic/localization sialoendoscopy. A guidewire can be passed through the working port of the endoscope, or the endoscope can be maintained in position, while a dissection is performed down to the stone so that it can be removed. For the intraoral technique, for the removal of the submandibular stones, attention should be focused on the lingual nerve dissection and the appropriate retraction of the nerve to prevent a permanent sensory change to the tongue. In the extraoral approach, only blunt dissection should be used to prevent damage to the facial nerve. The parotid capsule also should be closed tightly to prevent sialocele formation.

Techniques: Lithotripsy

Lithotripsy is the fragmentation of a calculus within the body of tissue, followed at once by the displacement of the fragments from the saliva or irrigation fluid out of the duct or physical removal of the calculus remnants. It formerly was done only surgically but can now be done by various noninvasive methods. The methods of lithotripsy are designated by the type of energy that fragments the stone, and whether the energy is introduced to the stone directly (intracorporeal) or extraorally (extracorporeal).

Intracorporeal Techniques

Mechanical fragmentation

Mechanical fragmentation can be achieved using grasping or crushing forceps. This can be done under direct observation using a sialoendoscope, or it can be performed in a blinded fashion. The blinded fashion is not recommended because of the potential of damage to adjacent tissue structures. Difficulty with this technique can occur if the density of the stone prevents the stone from fracturing. If too much force is used, the grasping forcing can be damaged. Larger fragments are removed using grasping forceps, or wire stone removal baskets. The small remaining granules will be expressed in the saliva, and patients usually report an occasional sandy consistency to their saliva over the next 30 to 60 days.

Intracorporeal laser lithotripsy

Erbium: yttrium-aluminum-garnet laser Erbium: yttrium-aluminum-garnet Er: YAG lasers emit an infrared light with a wavelength of 2940 nm, which is absorbed strongly by water. Because of the fluid environment that is present in sialoendoscopy, the use of this type of laser is limited but relatively safe. To perform lithotripsy with the ER: YAG, a probe must be in close contact with the sialolith.

An erbium fiber delivery system consists of 99.9% pure silver tubes with polished sapphire rod tips. This device is able to deliver pulsed energy to the stone, with stone fragmentation rates of about 1.8 mm³/s. Unfortunately, following use, pitting of sapphire rod occurred, causing a degradation of fiber transmission. Because of this limitation, the use of erbium laser for sialolithotripsy is not ideal at this time.[12]

Holmium: yttrium-aluminum-garnet (HO: YAG) laser The holmium: yttrium-aluminum-garnet HO: YAG laser is a thermal laser that uses a 2150 nm wavelength of light. The energy is delivered in multiple pulses through low water density quartz fibers. The energy available at the tip of the holmium laser does not depend on the diameter of the fiber. The mechanism of stone fragmentation is based on a plasma-induced shock wave that is generated following the creation of a water channel between the fiber tip and the salivary stone. Soft tissue damage can and does occur with the HO: YAG laser, although it is limited in its nature. The amount of soft tissue damage is directly proportional to the amount of pulses that are needed to perform the lithotripsy. The HO: YAG laser disrupts the salivary stone into fine particles, as opposed to fragmentation of the stone. This is advantageous, because larger fragments created from other techniques can become lodged within the gland or the duct. The disadvantage to this is that it takes a considerable amount of time, limiting its use to smaller sialoliths.

Pneumatic lithotripsy

Pneumatic lithotripsy is performed by inserting a rigid probe through or lateral to the endoscope. The central unit is connected to a high pressure air system that delivers a 3 atm shock, 12 and 15 times a second, to the distal end of the semirigid metal probe. The energy is generated by the pressured air propelling a pellet at the distal wall of the hand piece, which is in contact with the stone. This energy is transmitted directly to the stone, which results in a fracture of the stone. Multiple fragments then are removed using basket or forceps techniques. The limitation of this technique is that the probe for this device is not compatible with the current sialoendoscope. Reported cases used a pediatric urethroscope, which generally is not used secondary to its relatively large diameter.[13]

Extracorporeal lithotripsy

Extracorporeal lithotripsy is performed by applying externally applied, focused, multiple high-intensity acoustic pulses, termed shock waves, in the direction of the sialolith. A shock wave is characterized by a very rapid pressure increase in the transmission medium. The shock waves from the lithotripter are delivered through an aqueous gel into the soft tissue. Passage of the shock wave through the soft tissue does not diminish the energy wave significantly. At both the entrance and exit of the stone, the potential energy of the shock wave is transformed into kinetic energy, causing both compressive and tensile forces and cavitation of the stone, causing fissuring in the stone, which after multiple shocks, results in to stone fragmentation. Factors that influence the likelihood of fragmentation are the size, microcrystalline structure, and architecture of the stone.[14] These fragments are removed if they are large, or are washed out

in the saliva. Best results are found in calculi that are 7 mm or less in size.[9]

Extracorporeal lithotripters generally have a gel-filled contact, termed a therapy head, which is placed either under the neck for submandibular stones, or for parotid stones, overlying the parotid gland. The shock wave pulse is transmitted through the soft tissues of the neck or the skin overlying the parotid gland to fractionate the stone. Acoustic damage is a possible concern, but there is little evidence to support this occurrence.[15]

PERIOPERATIVE MANAGEMENT

Sialoendoscopy should be considered a contaminated technique, because it is introducing an instrument from a nonsterile location (the mouth) into sterile organs. This being said, an appropriate antibiotic should be given to the patient before commencing surgery. The most effective antibiotic that should be administered has not been determined. At the author's institution, intravenous Unasyn (ampicillin sodium/sulbactam sodium) 3.0 g or clindamycin 600 mg is used, because of broad coverage, particularly of gram-positive cocci, which predominate in salivary gland bacterial infections. To decrease postsurgical edema, an intravenous corticoid steroid also is administered. A surgical drain/removable stent should be placed for 2 to 4 weeks to prevent adhesion formation with the duct.

POSTOPERATIVE MANAGEMENT

Postoperative antibiotics generally are administered, because of the possibility of the contamination of the gland. Additionally, the salivary gland generally is inflamed following surgery, and it takes 2 to 4 weeks, as determined by scintigraphy, for the gland to return to normal function. Without a steady salivary flow, retrograde migration of bacteria can occur.

POSSIBLE COMPLICATIONS

Potential complications can be divided into seven categories: (1) inability to remove the stone or an associated fragment, (2) postoperative infection, (3) change in peripheral nerve function, (4) intraductal adhesion formation, (5) subglossal scar band formation, (6) sialocele formation, and (7) ranula formation.

Inability to Remove Stone or Retention of Sialolith Fragments

When fragmenting large stones, or when removing brittle stones, sometimes fragments can be displaced and not located. This can be because the fragment is small and is displaced into a tertiary system, or it can occur later in the procedure, when the tissue has become edematous from extravasated irrigation fluid. There are three possible outcomes to this:

> The small stone or fragments will be expelled from the salivary gland with expressed saliva
>
> They can become encapsulated into the gland proper, without causing recurrent infections or obstruction.
>
> They can be the source of further obstruction and/or infections. If this, either a second sialolithectomy or a sialadenectomy must be performed.

Postoperative Infections

As covered in postoperative management, postoperative infections, although rare, need to be treated with antibiotics, either oral or intravenous, if indicated, and in the case of abscess formation, incision and drainage.

Change in Peripheral Nerve Function

As discussed previously, lingual nerve neurosensory dysfunction can occur from manipulation of the lingual nerve or facial nerve during parotid surgery. Following sialoendoscopic-assisted removal of a salivary stone, it is not uncommon to have some paresthesia of the tongue, which generally resolves in 1 to 3 months. In the parotid gland, if the appropriate dissection is used, facial muscle weakness is most likely a neuropraxia from the blunt dissection or a retraction pressure.

Intraductal Adhesion Formation

If intraductal adhesions occur, lysis is recommended. Because these adhesions are generally immature, they can be disrupted with lacrimal probes, a balloon dilator, or with a smaller diameter sialoendoscope. A postlysis/dilation stent should be placed once again for 2 to 4 weeks.

Subglossal Scar Band Formation

In intraoral sialoendoscopic-assisted sialolithectomy, the floor of the mouth is incised. Although primary closure is performed, a subglossal scar band can occur, which can cause a limitation of movement of the tongue, or the deviation of the tongue to the banded side. In the author's. institution, if this occurs, the scar band generally is lysed, and a mucoplasty is performed, approximately 4 weeks postoperatively, using a CO_2 laser, which results in the resolution of the limitation of movement within 1 to 2 weeks.

Sialocele Formation

In performing an extraoral removal of a parotid stone, or following perforation of Stenson's duct during the surgery, it is possible that a sialocele can occur, with extraoral drainage. This usually resolves with either high-pressure wrappings, closure of the parotid capsule, or a combination of both.

Ranula Formation

During submandibular stone formation, the sublingual duct as it joins the submandibular gland, or the sublingual gland itself can be damaged, and a ranula can occur. Uncovering the ranula should be performed. If resolution does not occur, removal of the sublingual gland may be indicated.

SUMMARY

Sialoendoscopy has become an excellent technique for treating various salivary gland diseases. Its role in salivary gland sparing surgery is essential, and over time, should decrease the number of sialadenectomies for the treatment of sialolithiasis, salivary strictures, and some patients who have chronic salivary gland infections. Its use for managing salivary oncology should be approached with caution. In other cases, consideration for the sparing of the salivary gland should be given greater consideration. Patients are living longer with the aid of medications that secondarily cause hyposalivation. Decreased salivary production may result in cervical dental caries, candidiasis, erosion and ulceration of mucosal tissues, dysgeusia, dysphagia, and effects that can cause a significant decrease in the quality of life.[16] The removal of each gland causes a decrease in salivary function of 15% to 35%, which in conjunction with pharmaceutical induced hyposalivation can result in a disastrous degeneration in the oral health and quality of life of patients.

REFERENCES

1. Gundlach P, Scherer H, Hopf J, et al. [Endoscopic-controlled laser lithotripsy of salivary calculi. In vitro studies and initial clinical use]. HNO 1990;38(7): 247–50 [in German].
2. Konigsberger R, Feyh J, Goetz A, et al. [Endoscopic controlled laser lithotripsy in the treatment of sialolithiasis]. Laryngorhinootologie 1990;69(6):322–3 [in German].
3. Katz P. [Endoscopy of the salivary glands]. Ann Radiol (Paris) 1991;34:110–3 [in French].

4. Konigsberger R, Feyh J, Goetz A, et al. Endoscopically controlled electrohydraulic intracorporeal shock wave lithotripsy (EISL) of salivary stones. J Otolaryngol 1993;22(1):12–3.

5. Arzoz E, Santiago A, Garatea J, et al. Removal of a stone in Stensen's duct with endoscopic laser lithotripsy: report of case. J Oral Maxillofac Surg 1994; 52(12):1329–30.

6. Nahlieli O, Neder A, Baruchin AM. Salivary gland endoscopy: a new technique for diagnosis and treatment of sialolithiasis. J Oral Maxillofac Surg 1994; 52(12):1240–2.

7. Marchal F, Becker M, Dulguerov P, et al. Interventional sialendoscopy. Laryngoscope 2000;110:318–20.

8. Zenk J, Hosemann WG, Iro H. Diameters of the main excretory ducts of the adult human submandibular and parotid gland: a histologic study. Oral Surg Oral Med Oral Pathol Oral Radiol Endod 1998; 85(5):576–80.

9. Ngu RK, Brown JE, Whaites EJ, et al. Salivary duct strictures: nature and incidence in benign salivary obstruction. Dentomaxillofac Radiol 2007;36(2): 63–7.

10. Jacobi CA, Bonjer HJ, Puttick MI, et al. Oncologic implications of laparoscopic and open surgery. Surg Endosc 2002;16(3):441–5.

11. Nahlieli O, Shacham R, Shlesinger M, et al. Juvenile recurrent parotitis: a new method of diagnosis and treatment. Pediatrics 2004;114(1):9–12.

12. Raif J, Vardi M, Nahlieli O, et al. An Er: YAG laser endoscopic fiber delivery system for lithotripsy of salivary stones. Lasers Surg Med 2006;38(6):580–7.

13. Arzoz E, Santiago A, Esnal F, et al. Endoscopic intracorporeal lithotripsy for sialolithiasis. J Oral Maxillofac Surg 1996;54(7):847–50.

14. Glasgow RE. Chapter 63 – treatment of gallstone disease. In: Feldman M, Friedman LS, Brandt LJ, editors. Feldman: Sleisenger & Fordtran's gastrointestinal and liver disease. 8th edition. Philadelphia: Saunders Elsevier; 2006. p. 1421–2.

15. Fritsch MH. Decibel levels during extracorporeal lithotripsy for salivary stones. J Laryngol Otol 2008; 122(12):1305–8.

16. Turner M, Jahangiri L, Ship JA. Hyposalivation, xerostomia and the complete denture: A systematic review. J Am Dent Assoc 2008;139(2):146–50.

Non-HIV Viral Infections of the Salivary Glands

Andrea Schreiber, DMD[a],*, Gabriel Hershman, DDS[b]

KEYWORDS

- Mumps • Paramyxovirus • Parotitis • Complications
- Vaccines • Epidemic

The viral organism that first comes to mind when considering non-HIV viral infections of the salivary glands, is the mumps virus. The derivation of the term "mumps" is often attributed to the Danish word *mompen*, meaning garbled speech, a common manifestation of the salivary gland swelling associated with the infection. Alternatively, it is described as deriving from the Old English word meaning "lumps" or "bumps." Although the incidence of mumps has been reduced significantly by the introduction of the mumps vaccine in 1967, sporadic outbreaks continue to be reported. Other non-HIV viruses detected in saliva or known to affect the salivary glands include Epstein-Barr virus (EBV), cytomegalovirus (CMV), human herpes simplex virus (HHSV-8), hepatitis C virus (HCV), human papilloma virus (HPV), cocksackie, influenza, and echovirus. Knowledge regarding the pathophysiology and sequelae of these viruses on the salivary glands remains somewhat limited to date.

The primary focus of this chapter is covered in two main subsections: Paramyxovirus-induced parotitis (MUMPS) and Other viral salivary gland infections.

PARAMYXOVIRUS-INDUCED PAROTITIS (MUMPS)
History

Although acute bacterial and viral infections are the most common ailments to affect salivary glands, infections of the salivary glands may, on occasion, also be caused by parasites and fungi. However, mumps remains the most common viral disease of the salivary glands. Mumps is an acute, self-limiting, contagious infectious disease that is most commonly characterized by bilateral non-suppurative parotid swelling, although all salivary glands may be involved.[1]

Before the introduction of a vaccine in 1967, more than 90% of school-age children were reported to have been exposed to mumps, and mumps epidemics were reported to have occurred in cycles every few years. In an epidemic in the early 1940s, an incidence of 250 of 100,000 was reported. This incidence declined sharply to 76 of 100,000 one year after the release of the live mumps vaccine and to about 1 case per 100,000 people some 20 years later. The decline in mumps incidence has been attributed to the increased usage of the mumps vaccine. In 1996, the Centers for Disease Control and Prevention (CDC) reported only 751 cases of mumps nationwide or about 1 case for every 5,000,000 people.

Signs and Symptoms

The mumps virus is contracted most frequently in childhood and adolescence, with more than 85% of cases occurring in persons under the age of 15 years.[2] The clinical presentation is frequently mild; not infrequently patients may be asymptomatic.[1] Adults are rarely infected because of immunity from vaccination or childhood exposure.[3]

The mumps virus is a paramyxovirus from the influenza and Newcastle groups. Like measles, it is a single-stranded RNA virus. Humans are its only natural host. Infection follows exposure through the upper respiratory tract by droplets, aerosol, direct contact, or fomites. After an

---

[a] Department of Oral and Maxillofacial Surgery, New York University College of Dentistry, New York, NY, USA
[b] Department of Oral and Maxillofacial Surgery, New York University-Bellevue Hospital Center, New York, NY, USA
* Corresponding author.
E-mail address: andrea.schreiber@nyu.edu (A. Schreiber).

Oral Maxillofacial Surg Clin N Am 21 (2009) 331–338
doi:10.1016/j.coms.2009.04.003

incubation period of several weeks an active viremia develops. Typically, patients present with prodromal symptoms of fever, malaise, and headache. Approximately 24 hours later, glandular swelling, tenderness, and associated earache can occur. Individuals are considered to be contagious immediately before, or at the onset of, glandular swelling. Resolution of symptoms generally occurs within 10 days.[4] Clinical findings include an enlarged, firm gland (see **Fig. 1**). Erythema and warmth to touch are not common. The overwhelming majority of cases involve both glands. Imaging studies are not routine but when performed show diffuse glandular inflammation.[3]

A logistic regression of the 2006 Iowa mumps outbreak indicated that the probability of mumps shedding after the onset of symptoms decreases rapidly. As a result of this analysis, the mumps isolation recommendation of the American Academy of Pediatrics has been changed from 9 days to 5 days. The virus can be isolated from the saliva for up to a week before symptoms develop, and it is considered most contagious within 2 days of development of parotitis.[5]

The peak incidence of mumps is in preschool, early elementary school age populations. It is characterized by an incubation of up to 3 weeks (mean, 18 days), with a prodrome of malaise, fever, anorexia, headache and myalgia followed by salivary gland pain and swelling, earache, trismus, and dysphagia.

Diagnosis, during an epidemic, is made on the basis of clinical findings, but viral serology is necessary to confirm the diagnosis of viral sialadenitis. Laboratory confirmation is made by testing for antibodies to mumps S and V antigens and to the hemagglutination antigen.[6] Complement fixing antibodies are detected after viral exposure. Soluble antibodies appear within the final week of infection and last for several months after infection. Soluble antibodies, directed at the nucleoprotein core of the virus, are therefore associated with recent vaccination or active infection. Viral antibodies, directed at the surface hemagglutinin, persist for years after exposure. Antibody titers to nonparamyxoviruses are also detectable.[2]

Treatment

The treatment of mumps is palliative and supportive and includes rest, hydration, and antipyretics. Arguably, the most significant advancement in the management of mumps has been the development of the live attenuated virus, which is frequently administered with the measles and rubella vaccines (MMR). The Jeryl Lynn vaccine, which is exclusively used in the United States, is considered to be both safe and efficacious.[3]

Complications

Complications of mumps, including, orchitis, oophoritis, mastitis, meningioencephalitis, pancreatitis, and deafness, are only infrequently reported. Before the widespread use of the mumps vaccine, the virus was a common cause of meningitis and encephalitis worldwide and in up to 36% of reported cases in the United States.[7] An association between mumps and the rapid onset of childhood diseases has also been reported.[6]

Complications relate to the systemic nature of the disease and the affinity of the virus for exocrine glands via hematogenous spread. Orchitis is the most frequent complication—occurring in up to 30% of affected boys, whereas oophoritis is reported in 5% of affected girls. Mumps orchitis usually resolves with palliative treatment in less than 10 days. Interferon α2a is recommended for patients with postpubertal mumps to prevent testicular atrophy and infertility.[1] Aseptic meningitis is reported in up to 10% of patients, whereas pancreatitis is found in fewer than 5% of patients. Sensorineral hearing loss is rare, but when it occurs, it is profound and often permanent.[3]

Numerous viruses exhibit tropism for the central nervous system (CNS), which can be manifested by a variety of clinical signs and symptoms. Spread to the CNS is accomplished by either hematogenous or neuronal routes. According to the CDC, more than 100,000 cases of aseptic meningitis are reported annually. Since the introduction of widespread vaccination programs, mumps account for a very small number of these cases. Meningitis is characterized by inflammation of the membranes surrounding the spinal cord and the brain, whereas encephalitis is characterized by infection of the brain tissue. Both meningitis and encephalitis

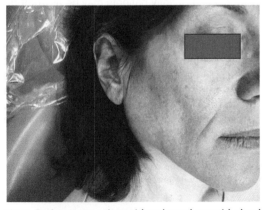

Fig. 1. Patient presenting with enlarged parotid gland associated with paramyxovirus-induced parotitis. (*Courtesy of* Michael D. Turner DDS, MD, FACS, New York, NY.)

may present with fever, headaches, and nuchal rigidity. Meningitis develops in up to 10% of patients with mumps parotitis, which is characterized by fever, headache, nausea and vomiting. Seizures are rarely reported. Examination of the cerebrospinal fluid (CSF) for virus-specific serologies is recommended, and mumps, rabies, CMV and nonpolio enteroviruses may be cultured from CSF. Enteroviruses, HHSV, and arboviruses (mosquito and tick mediated) account for the majority of meningitis and encephalitis cases. Hypoglycorrhachia is common with CMV and mumps infection but not with other, more common, viral infections. Mumps-related meningitis is considered in cases of unvaccinated children and adolescents, especially in the late winter and early spring months when arboviruses are less likely to be encountered. Most patients recover from mumps meningitis without long-term sequelae.

Meningioencephalitis can result in significant neurologic deficit and, rarely, death.[1] Meningioencephalitis has an occurrence rate of 2.5/100,000 cases. Mumps-related encephalitis, although exceedingly rare (approximately 0.2% of cases) and generally mild with low mortality, is associated with more significant CNS sequelae including seizures, persistent headaches, deafness, and optic atrophy.[8]

In 2002, Khubchandani and colleagues[8] reported the development of a case of mumps-related bilateral neuroretinitis characterized by decreased visual acuity and color perception and visual field deficits.

Mumps thyroiditis is another unusual complication of the infection. It may occur up to months after the development of parotitis and has not been reported to occur in the absence of or before the clinical manifestation of parotitis. Clinical features include gland enlargement accompanied by dysphagia and hoarseness. Most cases resolve spontaneously without long-term effects, although some cases of recurrent exacerbations and hypothyroidism have been reported.[9]

In 2006, Ishida and colleagues[10] reported three cases of mumps presenting with progressive edema and laryngoscopy-confirmed supraglottic edema and airway obstruction. The patients were treated with corticosteroids or tracheostomy. Dyspnea was attributed to swelling of parotid and submandibular glands bilaterally.

Outbreaks

In 1989 an outbreak of mumps in Kansas occurred among primary and secondary school students who had a vaccination history of 97%. The highest population of occurrence was in the junior high school population, especially in students who had received only one dose of vaccine. The outbreak was attributed to a combination of factors including vaccine failure and failure to vaccinate on a two-dose schedule.[11]

The largest outbreak of mumps since the 1988 inception of a vaccination program occurred in the United Kingdom in 1996. The outbreak involved children born between 1982 and 1983, who did not receive the vaccine. Salivary IgM was utilized to confirm recent mumps. It is thought that the outbreak was caused by diminished natural exposure in this nonvaccinated population. A targeted immunization program was contemplated for this age group of individuals.[12]

An outbreak of mumps in primary school-aged children occurred in Belgium in 1995 through 1996. An investigation of possible etiologies included inadequate vaccination schedule, primary or secondary vaccine failure, or low vaccination coverage. Primary vaccine failure refers to individuals who do not undergo serologic conversion after vaccination. Secondary vaccine failure refers to the occurrence of the disease in individuals who showed serologic conversion after vaccination. The study determined that the most probable reason for the outbreak was low vaccination coverage in that particular geographic area. At the time, Belgium had a two-dose vaccination schedule with the second dose at 11 years instead of the 4- or 5-year-old age group, common in the United States. The closer-spaced dosage regimen is thought to be preferable because it offers better control of the diseases, higher vaccination coverage, and a smaller number of susceptible individuals.[13]

A two-fold increase in the number of mumps outbreaks was noted in England and Wales in 2004 compared with 2003. This followed a few prior years of more modest elevations. The cohort of individuals most affected were young adults born before 1988 who would have been too old to have received MMR when it was first introduced. Consideration was given to offering two doses of MMR to this age group at high risk, especially those entering university.[14]

In 2006, the U.S. Centers for Disease Control and Prevention received reports of more than 500 cases of possible mumps in Iowa. The total number of reported cases (more than 2500) represented a greater than 10-fold increase over prior years. Most of the reported patients in Iowa were of college age, and more than 80% had received two doses of mumps-containing vaccine in childhood: 6% had not been vaccinated, and 12% had received one vaccination. The strain of mumps identified in this cohort was the same as that present in the vaccine, which therefore should have been protective. The same strain had been identified in many cases in the United Kingdom, but most of those cases occurred in unvaccinated individuals[15,16] Mumps outbreaks in Canada and the United States in 2005 through 2006 accounted for more than 10,000 reported cases. The same strain (genotype G) has been identified in all isolates.[17]

Some studies of vaccinated populations affected by mumps outbreaks indicate a potential that the longer the time from vaccination, the greater the risk for mumps to have occurred. However, there is no definitive proof of a decline in protection with increasing age or time from vaccination.[18]

Mumps virus detection rates are higher from saliva than from urine or throat swabs. The use of reverse transcriptase polymerase chain reaction has enabled the identification of up to 12 virus sequences that belong to three main lineage groups. The cocirculation of multiple strains or the accumulation of sufficient point mutations may be responsible for periodic outbreaks.[19]

Vaccines

Despite the widespread use of an effective vaccine, mumps has yet to be eradicated. The reasons for this have not been clearly elucidated. Currently, 5 different vaccine strains are in use worldwide. The Jeryl Lynn strain is currently the only one in use in the United States. It has a strong safety profile and has never been associated with the development of aseptic meningitis, as other vaccine strains have. The other strains, the Urabe, the Rubini, the Lenigrad-Zagreb, and the Leningrad-3 strains are all either less effective or less safe than the Jeryl Lynn vaccine.[17] An outbreak of mumps in Scandinavia in 1996 was attributed to the low efficacy of the Rubini vaccine in comparison to the Jeryl Lynn vaccine, which induces a stronger humoral response than the other vaccine strains.[20]

Evidence of mumps protection is presumed in individuals born before 1957, individuals who have received two doses of mumps-containing vaccine, individuals with a documented history of mumps, and individuals with titer evidence of immunity. Current recommendations from the Centers for Disease Control and Prevention (CDC), the American Academy of Pediatrics, and the American Academy of Family Physicians includes a first vaccine dose after age 12 months followed by a second dose between the ages of 4 and 6 years. Recommendations for health care workers are the administration of two doses of vaccine for individuals without a history of vaccination or proof of immunity. Updated recommendations in 2006 stress the importance of vaccination in college-aged individuals.[21]

The 1987 and 2006 mumps outbreaks in the Midwestern United States underscored the importance of ensuring the immunity of health care workers. Health care workers without documented immunity may not be allowed to work for several weeks after exposure. Serologic evidence of immunity or documented evidence of vaccination is therefore currently recommended by the Advisory Committee on Immunization Practices of the CDC.[22]

Vaccine efficacy is reported to be approximately 97%. A disparity between controlled clinical trials and field studies has been documented, with field studies reporting 75% to 95% efficacy. Additionally, antibody levels induced by natural infections appear to be higher than those induced by vaccination. The duration of immunity is not known, but epidemiologic studies report continuing immunity for more than 30 years.[23]

Mechanisms of vaccine failure may relate to delay in use after reconstitution of the vaccine, improper storage and handling of the vaccine, and settings that facilitate transmission of shed viral particles (eg, school, camp). Concerns about waning immunity have been raised but remain to be proven.[24]

Outbreaks continue to be reported worldwide, even in vaccinated individuals. Korea, which has a robust immunization program, reports periodic outbreaks in school-aged children regularly every few years. In an effort to determine the reasons for vaccine failure, Park and Nam[24] utilized IgG avidity testing to distinguish between primary and secondary vaccine failure. Assessment of IgG antibody avidity was found to be a reliable tool for differentiating between primary and secondary vaccine failure. The test is based on the fact that in primary infection, the IgG antigen/antibody bond is weak (low avidity), whereas in secondary infection, the rapid antibody response is characterized by a stronger bond (high avidity). Their results suggested that secondary failure may be the cause of periodic mumps epidemics in vaccinated populations. They suggest that a booster vaccine may be indicated in adolescent populations.[24] In 2000, Takahishi and colleagues[4] found that several genotypes of mumps appear to be cocirculating and may be the cause of the episodic outbreaks.

In 1998, Narita and colleagues conducted an analysis of mumps vaccine failure by means of avidity testing for mumps virus-specific IgG. They found this to be superior to IgM in distinguishing primary and secondary failure. It is currently not clear if a booster immunization would facilitate avidity maturation.[25]

Currently no postexposure prophylaxis for mumps is available, and little is known about mumps in the immunocompromised host. Although MMR is conventionally contraindicated in immunocompromised patients, it is recommended for asymptomatic HIV-positive children. Mumps in pregnancy does not seem to be associated with congenital deformities.[26]

The administration of a second-dose mumps vaccine in school-aged children in the United States was initiated in 1990. This was followed by a dramatic decrease in reported cases until the outbreak of 2006. The outbreak was first reported in Iowa and then centered around eight adjacent states with a total of more than 6500 reported cases. The highest percentage was reported in the 18- to24-year-old age group; 84% of these patients reported receiving two doses of vaccination.

Future directions of research will focus on whether waning immunity indeed exists and, if so, whether administration of a second dose of vaccine at a later age or whether administration of a third dose will provide more reliable immunity.[27]

OTHER VIRAL SALIVARY GLAND INFECTIONS
Epstein-Barr Virus

Epstein-Barr virus (EBV) is a complex DNA virus member of the herpesviridae family. EBV, like other members of this family establishes lifelong infection with periodic reactivation and shedding. Salivary glands can be chronically infected with EBV, and saliva is the only bodily fluid shown to shed viral particles. EBV is associated with infectious mononucleosis, nasopharyngeal carcinoma, Burkitt's lymphoma, and chronic neurasthenia syndrome.[28]

There is circumstantial evidence linking EBV to Sjögren's syndrome, an autoimmune disorder characterized by lymphocytic infiltration of the salivary and lacrimal glands. Immunohistochemical studies have found that the salivary duct epithelium is the primary site of EBV replication. It is hypothesized that the inflammation of Sjögren's syndrome could be caused by the breakdown or lack of immune response normally seen in the ductal epithelium. However, no increased EBV viral load has been detected in Sjögren's syndrome patients, nor has a positive association of EBV and the etiology of Sjögren's syndrome been confirmed.[29]

Fox and colleagues[30] investigated whether EBV plays a role in the pathogenesis of Sjögren's syndrome. DNA probes and monoclonal antibodies were used to detect evidence of viral gene products. Interest in EBV as a potential etiologic agent for Sjögren's syndrome is based on the finding of EBV replication within salivary glands, as well as the fact that these viruses (like other herpes viruses) remain latent in affected individuals. EBV is a potent stimulator of polyclonal B cells and can induce autoantibody synthesis including ANA and RF. Additional evidence for this association is the fact that several small RNA encoded by EBV are complexed with proteins precipitated by autoantibodies found in Sjögren's syndrome patients. An elevated content of EBV antigens and DNA was found in the salivary glands of these patients, but a mechanism for pathogenesis remains to be elucidated.[30]

Because a close association of EBV with the development of Burkitt's lymphoma, gastric carcinoma, and nasopharyngeal carcinoma has been documented by the presence of virally encoded antigens and EBV genomes, its potential association with other salivary gland tumors is under investigation. A study of the structure and expression of EBV DNA in these tumors may aid in determination of the role of EBV in the development of these malignancies.[31]

In a study by Tsai and colleagues,[32] 56 salivary gland carcinomas were evaluated to determine the role of EBV in their development. A close association between lymphoepithelioma-like carcinomas and EBV has been reported.[32] Wen and colleagues[33] reported that all cases of undifferentiated carcinomas and T-cell lymphomas in their study demonstrated EBV genomes, indicating the presence of EBV infection.

Hepatitis C

Because there are reports of histologic changes in the salivary glands of HCV-infected patients that resemble changes found in Sjögren's syndrome, Taliani and colleagues[34] sought to determine if HCV infects the salivary gland epithelial cells of patients with chronic hepatic HCV disease. No evidence of salivary gland HCV was detected in this study. Although low-level HCV RNA was detected in the saliva of some patients, it was hypothesized that this was caused by viral spillover from the blood of these patients, as all of these samples were from highly viremic patients. Currently, no association of HCV and Sjögren's syndrome has been found.

Salivary gland lesions characterized by lymphocytic infiltration of capillaries has been reported in approximately half of all HCV patients in this study. Lymphocytic sialadenitis resembling that found in Sjögren's syndrome is also sometimes reported in these patients. Other extrahepatic immunologic manifestations of chronic HCV infection include immune complex–mediated disorders, such as mixed cryoglobinemia and antitissue antibodies in the serum.[35]

In the absence of associated systemic autoimmune disease, patients with focal lymphocytic infiltration of exocrine glands and with clinical complaints of salivary and lacrimal dysfunction are considered to have Sjögren's syndrome. Although a viral etiology to Sjögren's syndrome has been postulated, findings, thus far, are inconclusive. A viral etiology would have some potential impact on medical management of these individuals, for example, interferon-α has been used to treat hepatic and extrahepatic effects of chronic HCV infection and has also been shown to have a beneficial effect on xerostomia in Sjogren's syndrome patients. Contrary to other studies, Garcia-Carrasco and colleagues[36] found HCV infection present in 14% of patients previously diagnosed with primary Sjögren's syndrome. The significance of this finding in determining the pathogenesis of the disease process is unclear.

Although chronic liver disease is the most heralded clinical manifestation of chronic HCV infection, almost 75% of patients develop an extrahepatic manifestation of the virus. Mixed cryoglobinemia has been associated with HCV in approximately 60% of patients. Mixed cryoglobinemia also has a high association with Sjögren's-like sialadenitis, and therefore, an association between Sjögren's syndrome and HCV has been postulated. Histologically, the lymphocytic infiltration in HCV appears to be pericapillary as opposed to the periductal infiltrate of Sjögren's syndrome. Clinical findings of xerostomia and xerophthalmia are less prevalent in HCV-infected patients than in those with primary Sjogren's syndrome. The term "Sjögren's syndrome secondary to chronic HCV infection" has been suggested to differentiate between the two entities. The pathogenesis of HCV-related sialadenitis is still unclear. Further research is necessary to determine if HCV causes a disease that mimics primary Sjögren's syndrome or if a causal relationship exists.[37]

Others

Because viruses are known to be involved in the etiology of both benign and malignant lesions in humans, and little is known about the etiology of salivary gland tumors, the possible involvement of HPV, EBV, CMV, and HHSV-8 in the development of salivary gland tumors continues to be investigated. The tumorigenic effects of viruses are thought to be mediated by proteins that prevent apoptosis by mimicking cell cycle regulatory proteins. In a study by Atula and colleagues,[38] 19 consecutive pleomorphic adenomas and 19 consecutive malignant salivary gland tumors were analyzed with polymerase chain reaction to detect evidence of viral DNA. EBV DNA was detected in two samples—a parotid lymphoma and a pleomorphic adenoma of the nasopharynx. HPV, CMV and herpesvirus DNA were not detected in any of the samples tested.[38]

Dalpa and colleagues[39] reported a high prevalence of HHSV-8 in Warthin's tumors in a study of 43 patients with the disease, suggesting a possible role of the virus in the pathogenesis of the tumor. Larger cohort studies are needed to determine the relationship, if any, between a variety of viruses and the pathogenesis of benign or malignant salivary gland tumors.[39]

Although mumps is most commonly caused by a paramyxovirus, a number of other viruses have been identified in acute viral parotitis. The nonparamyxoviruses, including influenza, parainfluenza, Cocksackie, echo, and lymphocytic choriomeningitic virus may account for multiple episodes of mumps in an individual patient.[2,40] CMV infections are generally mild with nonspecific findings and, unlike the mumps, occur primarily in adults.[41] EBV and HIV are detected in saliva but do not directly infect major salivary glands.

SUMMARY

Historically, the most significant non-HIV viral infection of salivary glands has been, and remains, mumps. Despite the widespread administration of mumps vaccines worldwide, sporadic outbreaks continue to be reported. Epidemiologic studies are invaluable in understanding the etiology of these outbreaks. Information gleaned from these studies, coupled with advances in immunology, virology, and DNA/RNA testing will hopefully result in the development of vaccination regimens to ensure eradication of the disease.

A number of other viruses are also known to affect the salivary glands. Some are known to replicate in the salivary glands and other may cause parotitis similar to, but clinically milder than, that caused by the mumps virus. Additional research is needed to determine the role, if any, of other viruses in the development of Sjögren's syndrome as well as benign and malignant tumors of the salivary glands.

REFERENCES

1. Casela R, Bernhard L, Lehmann K, et al. Mumps orchitis: report of a mini-epidemic. J Urol 1997;158: 2158–61.

2. Bradley PJ. Microbiology and management of sialadentitis. Curr Infect Dis Rep 2002;4:217–24.

3. McQuone SJ. Acute viral and bacterial infections of the salivary glands. Otolaryngol Clin North Am 1999;32:793–811.

4. Takahashi M, Nakayama T, et al. Single genotype of measles virus is dominant whereas several genotypes of mumps virus are co-circulating. J Med Virol 2000;62:278–85.

5. Polgreen PM, Bohnett LC, et al. The duration of mumps virus shedding after onset of symptoms. Clin Infect Dis 2008;46:1447–9.

6. Rice DH. Salivary gland disorders: neoplastic and nonneoplastic. Med Clin North Am 1999;83:197–217.

7. Peltola H. Infectious diseases: mumps vaccination and meningitis. Lancet 1993;341(8851):994–5.

8. Khubchandani R, Rane T, et al. Bilateral neuroretinitis associated with mumps. Arch Neurol 2002; 59(10):1633–6.

9. Parmar R, Bavdekar S, et al. Thyroiditis as a presenting feature of mumps. Pediatr Infect Dis J 2001; 20(6):637–8.

10. Ishida M, Fushiki H, et al. Mumps virus infection in adults: three cases of supra-glottic edema. Laryngoscope 2006;116(12):2221–3.

11. Hersh BS, Kent WK, et al. Mumps outbreak in a highly vaccinated population. J Pediatr 1991; 119(2):187–93.

12. Wehner H, Morris R, et al. A secondary school outbreak of mumps following the childhood immunization programme in England and Wales. Epidemiol Infect 2000;124:131–6.

13. Vandermeulen C, Roelants M, et al. Outbreak of mumps in a vaccinated child population: a question of vaccine failure? Vaccine 2004;22:2713–6.

14. Savage E, Ramsay M, et al. Mumps outbreaks across England and Wales in 2004: observational study. BMJ 2005;330:1119–20.

15. Gershman K, Rios S, et al. Centers for disease control, update: multi-state outbreak of mumps-United States, January 1 – 2006. MMWR Morb Mortal Wkly Rep 2006;55:559–63.

16. Hopkins RS, Jajosky RA, et al. Centers for disease control. summary of notifiable diseases – United States, 2003. MMWR Morb Mortal Wkly Rep 2005; 52:1–85.

17. Peltola H, Kulkarni P, et al. Mumps outbreaks in Canada and the United States: time for new thinking on mumps vaccines. Clin Infect Dis 2007;45:459–66.

18. Cohen C, White JM, et al. Vaccine effectiveness estimates, 2004–2005 mumps outbreak, England. Emerg Infect Dis 2007;13(1):12–7.

19. Afzal MA, Buchanan J, et al. RT-PCR based diagnosis and molecular characterization of mumps viruses derived from clinical specimens collected during the 1996 mumps outbreak in Portugal. J Med Virol 1997;52:349–53.

20. Germann D, Strohle A, et al. An outbreak of mumps in a population partially vaccinated with the Rubini strain. Scand J Infect Dis 1996;28:235–8.

21. Kancheria VS, Hanson IC. Mumps resurgence in the United States. J Allergy Clin Immunol 2006;118:938–41.

22. Andersen E. Mumps – new face on an old disease. AAOHN J 2006;54(10):425–6.

23. Sugg WC, Finger JA, et al. Field evaluation of live virus mumps vaccine. J Pediatr 1968;72:461–6.

24. Park DW, Nam HM, et al. Mumps outbreak in a highly vaccinated school population: assessment of secondary vaccine failure using IgG avidity measurements. Vaccine 2007;25:4665–70.

25. Narita M, Matsuzono Y, et al. Analysis of mumps vaccine failure by means of avidity testing for mumps virus-specific immunoglobulin G. Clin Diagn Lab Immunol 1998;5:799–803.

26. Gupta RK, Best J, et al. Mumps and the UK epidemic 2005. BMJ 2005;330:1132–5.

27. Dayan GH, Quinlisk P, et al. Recent resurgence of mumps in the United States. N Engl J Med 2008; 358(15):1580–9.

28. Jones JF, Strauss SE. Chronic Epstein-Barr virus infection. Annu Rev Med 1987;38:195–209.

29. Venables PJW, Chong GT, et al. Persistence of Epstein-Barr virus in salivary gland biopsies from healthy individuals and patients with Sjogren's syndrome. Clin Exp Immunol 1989;75:359–64.

30. Fox RI, Pearson G, et al. Detection of Epstein-Barr virus-associated antigens and DNA in salivary gland biopsies from patients with Sjogren's syndrome. J Immunol 1986;137:3162–8.

31. Raab-Traub N, Rajadurai P, et al. Epstein-Barr virus infection in carcinoma of the salivary gland. J Virol 1991;65:7032–6.

32. Tsai CC, Chen CL, et al. Expression of Epstein-Barr virus in carcinomas of major salivary glands: a strong association with lymphoepithelioma-like carcinoma. Hum Pathol 1996;27:258–62.

33. Wen S, Mizugaki Y, et al. Epstein-Barr virus infection in salivary gland tumors: lytic EBV infection in nonmalignant epithelial cells surrounded by EBV-positive T-lymphoma cells. Virology 1997;227:484–7.

34. Taliani G, Celestino D, et al. Hepatitis C infection of salivary gland epithelial cells: lack of evidence. J Hepatol 1997;26:1200–6.

35. Pawlotsky JM, Roudot-Thoraval F, et al. Extrahepatic immunologic manifestations in chronic Hepatitis C and Hepatitis C serotypes. Ann Intern Med 1995; 122:169–73.

36. Garcia-Carrasco M, Ramos M, et al. Hepatitis C virus infection in 'primary' Sjogren's syndrome: prevalence and clinical significance in a series of 90 patients. Ann Rheum Dis 1997;56:173–5.

37. Carazzo M. Oral diseases associated with hepatitis C virus infection. Part I: sialadenitis and salivary glands lymphoma. Oral Dis 2008;14:123–30.

38. Atula T, Grenman R, et al. Human papillomavirus, Epstein-Barr virus, human herpesvirus 8 and human cytomegalovirus involvement in salivary gland tumors. Oral Oncol 1998;34:391–5.

39. Dalpa E, Gourvas V, et al. High prevalence of human herpes virus 8 (HHV-8) in patients with Warthin's tumors of the salivary gland. J Clin Virol 2008;42: 182–5.

40. Silvers AR, Som PM. Salivary glands. Radiol Clin North Am 1998;36:941–66.

41. Ship JA. Diagnosing, managing and preventing salivary gland disorders. Oral Dis 2002;8:77–89.

HIV-associated Salivary Gland Disease

Rabie M. Shanti, DMD, Shahid R. Aziz, DMD, MD*

KEYWORDS
- Salivary gland • HIV • Lymphoepithelial cyst
- Parotid enlargement • HAART

The AIDS epidemic claimed approximately 2.5 to 3.0 million lives in 2006, and an estimated 5 million people acquired the human immunodeficiency virus (HIV), bringing the number of people globally living with the virus to 40 million.[1,2] More than 95% of individuals infected with HIV live in developing countries.[3] Head and neck lesions associated with HIV occur in more than 50% of HIV-positive patients and occur in approximately 80% of all patients with AIDS.[1] These lesions often present as early signs and symptoms of the afore-mentioned diseases. Head and neck lesions associated with HIV may lead to discomfort, dysfunction, or disability and are part of the management of HIV-infected patients to reduce morbidity and mortality.[4]

The most common salivary gland presentation in HIV-infected individuals is salivary gland swelling, which can be attributed to acute siala-denitis or with HIV-associated salivary gland disease (HIV-SGD). Clinically, HIV-infected patients have been shown to possess reduction in the salivary flow rates of the parotid, subman-dibular, and sublingual glands.[5–7] Furthermore, HIV-infected individuals are known to have saliva containing increased sodium, chloride, lysozyme, peroxidase, lactoferrin, and immuno-globulin A levels.[7] Interestingly, with the observed changes in the flow rate and composi-tion of saliva in the HIV population, there has only been one case reporting an association between sialolithiasis and HIV/AIDS.[8] HIV-SGD is observed in both adults and children infected with HIV; however, in children HIV-SGD is observed more commonly and might represent a slightly different disease process. The following chapter discusses the clinical symp-toms, pathogenesis, and treatment options for various pathologic entities of the salivary glands that are unique to the HIV population. A famil-iarity and understanding of these processes is of great value to the oral and maxillofacial surgeon who might encounter these patients.

PAROTID GLAND ENLARGEMENT

Parotid gland enlargement is reported to occur in approximately 1% to 10% of HIV-infected patients.[9–11] Enlargement of the parotid gland in HIV-infected patients is usually secondary to the development of benign lymphoepithelial cysts within the parotid gland. There exists significant debate with regard to the terminology used to describe parotid gland enlargement in the HIV population. For instance, numerous terms have been used to describe lymphatic parotid enlarge-ment in the HIV population, including benign lymphoepithelial cysts (BLEC), benign lymphoepi-thelial lesions (BLEL), cystic BLEL, AIDS-related lymphadenopathy, diffuse infiltrative lymphocy-tosis syndrome (DILS), cystic lymphoid hyper-plasia, and HIV-associated salivary gland disease. Although the differential diagnosis for parotid gland enlargement in the HIV population should include the disease processes that occur in the non-HIV population, the enlargement is usually secondary to BLEC. Parotid gland swelling has also been observed in patients on antiretrovi-ral therapy.[12]

Department of Oral and Maxillofacial Surgery, University of Medicine and Dentistry of New Jersey, New Jersey Dental School, 110 Bergen Street, Room B854, Newark, NJ 07103, USA
* Corresponding author.
E-mail address: azizsr@umdnj.edu (S.R. Aziz).

Oral Maxillofacial Surg Clin N Am 21 (2009) 339–343
doi:10.1016/j.coms.2009.04.002
1042-3699/09/$ – see front matter © 2009 Elsevier Inc. All rights reserved.

Benign Lymphoepithelial Cysts

BLEC are pathologic entities that are clinically and pathologically distinct from benign lymphoepithelial lesions. This is a rare manifestation of HIV disease that is characterized by bilateral parotid swelling, diffuse visceral CD8 lymphocytic infiltration, persistent CD8 lymphocytosis, and cervical lymphadenopathy.[13–16] BLEC has been reported to occur in the salivary glands or their lymph nodes, oral cavity (floor of mouth), tonsil, thyroid gland, pancreas, and juxtabronchial.[11,17–21] Before the era of HIV infections, BLEC of the parotid gland was a rare pathologic entity. The first case of BLEC of the parotid gland was reported by Hildebrandt in 1895, and, as of 1981, only 21 cases had been described. However, with the emergence of the HIV epidemic, the incidence of parotid gland BLEC has increased dramatically.[11,22,23] BLEC is now estimated to occur in 3% to 6% and 1% to 10% of HIV-positive adults and children, respectively. However, with the advent and widespread use of highly active antiretroviral therapy (HAART), the overall incidence of BLEC appears to be on the decline.[11] BLEC is so unusual in the HIV-negative population that cystic enlargement of the parotid gland warrants investigation clinical for the possibility of HIV infection.[24]

Similar to the controversy surrounding the aforementioned terminology used to describe parotid gland enlargement in the HIV population, there exists significant controversy as to the exact pathogenesis of BLEC. Multiple theories have been proposed as to the exact mechanism or pathologic events resulting in the development of these lesions and their being unique to HIV-infected individuals. What is known is that as the virus replicates, BLEC develop.[25] One popular postulate is that of parotid enlargement results from proliferation of the glandular epithelium that is trapped within the 5 to 10 embryologic-derived lymph nodes within the parotid gland.[17,26] It has also been postulated that lymphoid proliferation causes ductal obstruction resulting in ductal dilation that mimics a true cyst resulting in parotid enlargement.[26,27]

Histologically, lymphoepithelial cysts have been reported as appearing to arise in the parotid nodes usually with lymphoid hyperplasia surrounding the cystic spaces. The cysts are usually lined by squamous or cuboidal epithelium, with germinal centers and a dense infiltrate of lymphoidal cells.[26] Furthermore, these lesions usually display partial encapsulation by a fibrous capsule.[26] The lymphoid infiltrates in the HIV-associated lesion have features of AIDS-related generalized lymphadenopathy (eg, hyperplastic follicles with follicle lysis and depletion of mantle zones). Furthermore, studies have found that the histopathology from labial minor salivary gland tissue in HIV-infected individuals with parotid gland enlargement resembles that seen in Sjogren's syndrome.[28] However, the parotid lesions in the HIV-associated lesion appear more focal in comparison to the usual Sjogren's-associated lymphoepithelial lesions.

The clinical presentations of BLEC have been described to display bilateral (up to 80%) parotid swellings that are multiple (up to 90%), painless, soft, and maintain a slow, gradual progression in size. Unilateral parotid swellings have also been reported.[11,29] Rarely does BLEC involve any other salivary gland; however, there have been reports of submandibular gland involvement.[17] This lymphocytic infiltration may also result in xerostomia caused by destruction of acinar tissue.[28]

The diagnostic evaluation consists mainly of ultrasound scan, CT, and/or MRI. Ultrasound, CT, and MRI will find multiple thin walled cysts with diffuse cervical lymphadenopathy.[11] Any sign of cystic parotid gland enlargement on the aforementioned imaging modalities is an indication for HIV testing. In the pediatric patient, ultrasound scan has the advantages of lack of radiation exposure and not requiring sedation of the child.[30]

The management of parotid gland BLEC is not very well established, with differing opinion as to the optimal treatment algorithm. The treatment options for BLEC include the following: (1) close observation, (2) repeat aspiration, (3) antiretroviral medication, (4) sclerosing therapy, (5) radiation therapy, and (6) surgery.

With regard to the observation of BLEC, as previously mentioned, BLEC have a slow progression; therefore, any sudden increases in gland size warrant immediate investigation because of the risk of lymphomatous transformation. Fine-needle aspiration (FNA) has been shown to be an effective diagnostic tool for monitoring BLEC for the development of EBV-associated malignant B-cell lymphoma, of which these patients are at an increased risk.[28] Even though a relationship between BLEC and malignancy is not well documented, HIV patients have a higher incidence of malignant lymphoma, thus necessitating routine (every 6 months) follow-up. Thus, close monitoring for any suspicious clinical or radiographic changes should be done with special attention toward rapid growth of existing swelling.[11] In the case of rapid growth of BLEC, histopathologic analysis is required to rule out malignancy.[26] Monitoring it thus a reasonable option for asymptomatic lesions.

With the enlargement of the parotid and the cosmetic sequelae, some patients may seek more aggressive treatment, such as, aspiration. This is considered to be a quick, office-based procedure, and can be performed in conjugation with FNA.[24] The disadvantage of this treatment modality is that the majority of aspirated lesions will recur within a matter of weeks to months and subsequently continue to grow.[11,25]

Antiretroviral medications, such as, zidovudine (AZT) have been found to reduce or eliminate BLEC.[31] However, these studies have been limited and with varying results; thus, further studies are needed to determine the role of antiretroviral medication as a therapeutic option in the medical management of this disease process.

Sclerotherapy with doxycycline has shown significant promise for the treatment of BLEC.[19] Studies with short-term results have reported an average reduction in cyst size by 42% to 100%.[19,24] Although sclerotherapy is known for causing mild edema and/or tenderness, no serious complications (ie, facial nerve injury, infection) have been reported. Furthermore, if a surgical option is deemed necessary subsequently, parotidectomy does not appear more difficult.[11]

Radiation therapy is another therapeutic modality that has shown significant promise at reducing parotid gland size. Some investigators have advocated low-dose external radiation therapy as the standard of case for the treatment of BLEC.[11] Because of the ominous oral side effects of radiation therapy (ie, mucositis, xerostomia) and its subsequent use if the patient would go on to have lymphoma or Kaposi sarcoma, radiation therapy has been advocated by some investigators to be limited for palliation therapy in end-stage AIDS patients who have not responded to any other less-invasive therapeutic modalities.

Compared with the aforementioned therapeutic options, surgery is one that is rarely recommended for the treatment of BLEC. Because of the routine use of diagnostic imaging (eg, ultrasonography, CT, and MRI) and FNA, surgery is rarely indicated in the diagnosis of lesions that display minimal malignant potential. Furthermore, given the bilateral and progressive nature of the disease, and the risk of facial nerve injury, multiple surgical procedures would be needed to address treating the disease even after a superficial parotidectomy.[11] Enucleation has also been proposed as an alternative surgical option; however, the patient must be prepared for repeated enucleation procedures. Therefore, surgery is recommended only as the last resort when all other treatment options have failed (**Figs. 1**A, B and **2**A, B).

Antiretroviral Therapy–induced Parotid Swelling

Today, the accepted standard treatment for HIV is termed "highly active antiretroviral therapy" (HAART), which consists of a combination of reverse transcriptase inhibitors and protease inhibitors. Since the advent of HAART the morbidity and mortality rates associated with HIV infection have decreased significantly. This improvement in the morbidity and mortality rates in HIV patients unfortunately has been associated with systemic side effects and dramatic morphologic changes.[31] With regard to the latter, generalized wasting is a common manifestation in the HIV population. This syndrome is referred to as HIV-associated lipodystrophy. The most commonly affected regions of the body include the face, buttocks, and extremities. In contrast to the wasting phenomenon commonly observed with HAART, Mandel and Alfi[12] reported in 2008 a case series of two patients that had parotid swelling that was associated with long-term HAART. Maxillofacial CT imaging of both patients found depositions of subcutaneous fat in the paraparotid tissues in both patients. This accumulation of subcutaneous fat has been suggested to be an

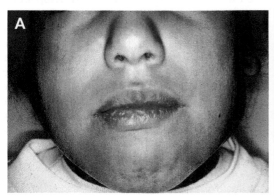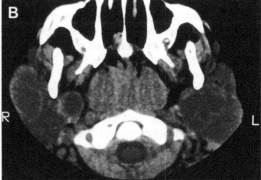

Fig. 1. (*A*) An 8-year-old HIV-positive boy with bilateral benign lymphoepithelial cysts. (*B*) CT scan of same patient shows bilateral BLEC (*Courtesy of* Louis Mandel, DDS, New York, NY).

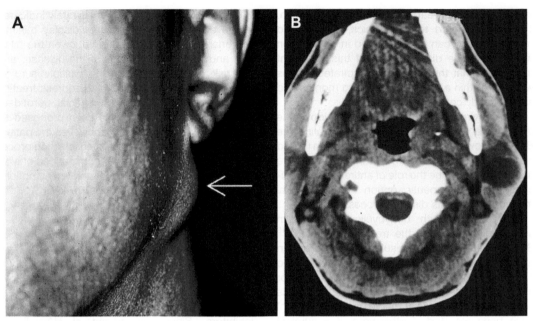

Fig. 2. (*A*) HIV-positive man with unilateral benign lymphoepithelial cyst. (*B*) CT scan of same patient shows unilateral BLEC (*Courtesy of* Louis Mandel, DDS, New York, NY).

indirect effect of subcutaneous fat wasting with the aforementioned visceral depots providing alternative sites for the storage of fat tissue lost in the peripheral areas. Today, HIV-associated lipodystrophy can be managed with a myriad of medical (eg, testosterone, anabolic steroids, growth hormone), pharmacologic (ie, metformin), and surgical therapies (eg, tumescent suction lipectomy, facial fillers, and autologous free fat). The aforementioned plastic surgery options can address the cosmetic issues related to HIV-associated lipodystrophy and have shown some success; however, control of the underlying process is best accomplished through diet and exercise.[12]

SALIVARY GLAND MALIGNANCY

Patients in later stages of immunocompromise in HIV/AIDS are known to have a higher incidence of malignancy, such as cutaneous squamous cell carcinoma or lymphoma. To date, there has been no clear link or correlation between HIV infection and increased rates of salivary gland malignancy. However, because of the histologic similarity between parotid duct and cutaneous epithelial cells it has been hypothesized that the human immunodeficiency virus may contribute to an increased risk of malignancy in infected patients. In 2008, Kim and colleagues[32] reported a case of primary squamous cell carcinoma confined to Stensen's duct in a patient with HIV. The patient

was subsequently treated with external beam radiation therapy at a dose of 5000 cGy over 6 weeks that was delivered to the primary site and the regional lymph nodes. The patient was known to be clinically disease free for 31 months after radiation therapy.

SUMMARY

We reviewed the clinical presentation, diagnostic evaluation, and treatment modalities for salivary gland enlargement in an HIV-infected population. Because this not an unusual finding in HIV-infected patients, it is of great significance to the oral and maxillofacial surgeon who is often faced with the challenge of managing these patients from a more diagnostic and treatment perspective.

REFERENCES

1. Yengopal V, Naidoo S. Do oral lesions associated with HIV affect quality of life? Oral Surg Oral Med Oral Pathol Oral Radiol Endod 2008;106(1):66–73.
2. UNAIDS. AIDS epidemic update December 2006. Geneva, Switzerland. Available at: http://www.unaids.org/. Accessed November 22, 2008.
3. Ranganathan K, Hemalatha R. Oral lesions in HIV infection in developing countries: an overview. Adv Dent Res 2006;19(1):63–8.
4. Adedigba MA, Ogunbodede EO, Jeboda SO, et al. Patterns of oral manifestations of HIV/AIDS among 225 Nigerian patients. Oral Dis 2008;14(4):341–6.

5. Yeh CK, Fox PC, Ship JA, et al. Oral defense mechanisms are impaired early in HIV-1 infection. J Acquir Immune Defic Syndr 1988;1:361–6.

6. Atkinson JC, Yeh CK, Oppenheim FG, et al. Elevation of salivary antimicrobial proteins following HIV-1 infection. J Acquir Immune Defic Syndr 1990;3: 41–8.

7. Capaccio P, Monforte A, Moroni M, et al. Salivary stone lithotripsy in the HIV patient. Oral Surg Oral Med Oral Pathol Oral Radiol Endod 2002;93(5): 525–7.

8. Ottaviani F, Galli A, Mothanje BL, et al. Bilateral parotid sialolithiasis in a patient with acquired immunodeficiency syndrome and immunoglobulin G multiple myeloma. Oral Surg Oral Med Oral Pathol Oral Radiol Endod 1997;83:552–4.

9. Morales-Aguirre JJ, Patino-Nino AP, Mendoza-Azpiri M, et al. Parotid cysts in children infected with human immunodeficiency virus. Arch Otolaryngol Head Neck Surg 2005;131:353–5.

10. Gaitan-Cepeda L, Morales J, Sanchez-Vargas L, et al. Prevalence of oral lesions in Mexican children with perinatally acquired HIV: association with immunologic status, viral load, and gender. AIDS Patient Care STDS 2002;16:151–6.

11. Dave SP, Pernas FG, Roy S. The benign lymphoepithelial cyst and a classification system for lymphocytic parotid gland enlargement in the pediatric HIV population. Laryngoscope 2007;117(1):106–13.

12. Mandel L, Alfi D. Drug-induced paraparotid fat deposition in patients with HIV. J Am Dent Assoc 2008;139(2):152–7.

13. Bachmeyer C, Dhote R, Blanche P, et al. Diffuse infiltrative CD8 lymphocytosis syndrome with predominant neurologic manifestations in tow HIV-infected patients responding to zidovudine. AIDS 1995;9: 1101–2.

14. Mandel L, Kim D, Uy C. Parotid gland swelling in HIV diffuse infiltrative CD8 lymphocytosis syndrome. Oral Surg Oral Med Oral Pathol Oral Radiol Endod 1998;85:565–8.

15. Schrot RJ, Adelman HM, Linden CN, et al. Cystic parotid gland enlargement in HIV disease: the diffuse infiltrative lymphocytosis syndrome. JAMA 1997;278:166–7.

16. Itescu S, Dalton J, Zhang H, et al. Tissue infiltration in a CD8 lymphocytosis syndrome associated with human immunodeficiency virus-1 infection has the phenotypic appearance of an antigenically drive response. J Clin Invest 1993;91:2216–25.

17. Elliott JN, Oertel YC. Lymphoepithelial cysts of the salivary glands: histologic and cytologic features. Am J Clin Pathol 1990;93:39–42.

18. Weidner H, Geisinger KR, Sterling RT, et al. Benign lymphoepithelial cysts of the parotid gland: a histologic, cytologic, and ultrastructural study. Am J Clin Pathol 1986;85:395–401.

19. Lustig RD, Lee KC, Murr A, et al. Doxycycline sclerosis of benign lymphoepithelial cysts in patients infected with HIV. Laryngoscope 1988;108:1199–205.

20. Favia G, Capodiferro S, Scivetti M, et al. Multiple parotid lymphoepithelial cysts in patients with HIV-infection: report of two cases. Oral Dis 2004;10: 151–4.

21. Brudnicki AR, Levin TL, Slim MS, et al. HIV-associated (non-thymic) intrathoracic lymphoepithelial cyst in a child. Pediatr Radiol 2001;31:603–5.

22. Morris MR, Moore DW, Shearer GL. Bilateral multiple benign lymphoepithelial cysts of the parotid gland. Otolaryngol Head Neck Surg 1987;97:87–90.

23. Huang RD, Pearlman S, Friedman WH, et al. Benign cystic vs. solid lesions of the parotid gland in HIV patients. Head Neck 1991;13:522–7.

24. Echavez MI, Lee KC, Sooy CD. Tetracycline sclerosis for treatment of benign lymphoepithelial cyst of the parotid gland in patients infected with human immunodeficiency virus. Laryngoscope 1994;104: 1499–502.

25. Mandel L, Reich R. HIV parotid gland lymphoepithelial cysts. Oral Surg Oral Med Oral Pathol 1992;74: 273–8.

26. Mandel L, Hong J. HIV-associated parotid lymphoepithelial cysts. J Am Dent Assoc 1999;130(4):528–32.

27. Ihrler S, Zeitz C, Riederer A, et al. HIV-related parotid lymphoepithelial cysts. Immunohistochemistry and 3-D reconstruction of surgical and autopsy material with special reference to formal pathogenesis. Virchows Arch 1996;429:139–47.

28. Patton LL, van der Horst C. Oral infections and other manifestations of HIV disease. Infect Dis Clin North Am 1999;13(4):879–900.

29. Al-Maawali AA, Chacko AP, Javad H, et al. HIV disease presenting as a unilateral parotid gland swelling. Indian J Pediatr 2008;75(10):1087–8.

30. Mayer M, Haddad J. Human immunodeficiency virus infection presenting with lymphoepithelial cysts in a six-year old child. Ann Otol Rhinol Laryngol 1996;105:242–4.

31. Shaha AR, DiMaio T, Webber C, et al. Benign lymphoepithelial lesions of the parotid. Am J Surg 1993;166:403–6.

32. Kim TB, Klein HZ, Glastonbury CM, et al. Primary squamous cell carcinoma of Stensen's duct in a patient with HIV: the role of magnetic resonance imaging and fine-needle aspiration. Head Neck 2009;31(2):278–82.

Diagnosis and Management of Pediatric Salivary Gland Infections

Ashish Patel, DDS, Vasiliki Karlis, DMD, MD, FACS*

KEYWORDS

- Salivary • Parotitis • JRP • Pediatric • Sialadenitis

PATHOPHYSIOLOGY/EPIDEMIOLOGY
Juvenile Recurrent Parotitis

Juvenile recurrent parotitis (JRP), formally called recurrent parotitis of childhood (RPC) is a chronic condition of childhood, which involves recurrent inflammation and infection of the salivary glands, commonly the parotids, without a definitive etiology. Most patients who are afflicted by this condition experience their first onset of symptoms between ages 3 and 6 years and have repeated bouts of parotitis until puberty.[1,2] Most studies report a slight male predominance in both prevalence and an earlier age of onset. In the majority of cases, this disease is self-limiting and does not progress after the onset of puberty. Although, by no means common, JRP is the most common inflammatory salivary gland disorder in the United States, the second most common parotid disease in children following viral mumps, worldwide.[3]

Imaging or histological examination reveals dilation of the distal ducts of the parotid gland and puntacte sialectasis, usually without obstruction, leading to chronic inflammation of the glandular parenchyma.[2,4,5] Many theories regarding the pathogenesis have been proposed, including the possibility of ascending oral bacteria through Stenson's duct, usually Gram-positive aerobes, causing chronic infection and dilation of the distal ducts.[1,2,6–8] Maynard proposed that recurrent episodes of parotid swelling are the end result in a sequence of the following events.

An initial low-grade inflammation of the gland and ductal epithelium, which is secondary to dehydration or impaired salivary flow, results in stricture and columnar metaplasia. The metaplastic epithelium increases mucous secretions, resulting in decreased clearance of the more viscous saliva and further reduction of salivary flow, predisposing the patient to recurrent parotitis.[9]

Decrease in salivary flow inevitably lowers the pH of the static secretions and predisposes the coagulation and accumulation of plasma proteins, such as lactoferrin and albumin, in the ductal system. This development creates another physical blockage of drainage acting synergistically with the lowered salivary flow rate. Increases in MMP-2, MMP-9, and kallikrein from affected glands suggest a chronic inflammatory response.[10,11]

Chronic inflammation of the gland leads to a lymphocytic periductal and intralobular infiltrate, which can have a cytotoxic effect on the glandular parenchyema. This can explain the edema and extravasation of secretions seen in JRP.[2]

A recent pilot study explored a possible link of JRP with dental malocclusion and masticatory apparatus strain. Another study showed marked improvement in parotid swelling and pain in nine out of 12 children aged 4–14 years, following a 6-month period of oral appliance/orthotic therapy for cases of malocclusion with concomitant JRP. Although this association may be caused by a spontaneous resolution of symptoms over the

Department of Oral and Maxillofacial Surgery, Advanced Education Program in OMS, NYU College of Dentistry, NYU Medical Center, 345 East 24th Street, NY, NY 10010, USA
* Corresponding author.
E-mail address: vk1@nyu.edu (V. Karlis).

Oral Maxillofacial Surg Clin N Am 21 (2009) 345–352
doi:10.1016/j.coms.2009.05.002
1042-3699/09/$ – see front matter © 2009 Published by Elsevier Inc.

6-month treatment period and the relatively short follow-up time, the authors suggest surrounding muscular spasticity may be an etiologic factor in the inflammatory response of the gland.[12]

No particular gene or inheritance pattern has been definitively identified in the etiology of this disease, but Reid and colleagues described an autosomal dominant pattern in JRP in a 1998 case series which showed a 75% (six out of eight) penetrance among siblings and parents.[3,13] This suggests some genetic factors may play a role in certain forms of the disease.

Clinically, acute exacerbations of JRP present with parotid edema and pain, usually without the presence of purulent exudate. This syndrome is usually self-limited and resolves within 2 weeks, but recurrences are frequent and can cause irreversible glandular damage. JRP usually presents unilaterally, but a bilateral parotid swelling, especially with one side being more severe, is not uncommon. Because flare-ups of JRP cause a brisk inflammatory response and can also be associated with bacterial or viral superinfection, systemic signs of malaise, leukocytosis, and fever may be present.[1,2,4,6–8,11]

The most common physical finding in exacerbations of JRP is an enlarged Stenson's papilla (which can be bilateral even in unilateral disease) with yellow plaques of coagulated proteins around the duct.[14–16] This finding is facilitated by palpation of the gland to express saliva from the duct. The gland itself will be indurated but painful to palpation. Patients may also suffer from xerostomia, which can induce other related conditions like halitosis, cervical dental demineralization and decay, and mild dysphagia.

Endoscopic examination usually reveals avascularity in the ductal layer of Stenson's duct with a characteristic white orifice as opposed to the microvascular net and pink appearance of healthy parotid duct tissue. This physical finding has also been demonstrated in adults with chronic salivary gland disease, but the immediate presentation of the physical findings on endoscopy, following juvenile parotid swelling, suggests that the hypovascularity is a causative or contributing agent to the disease process rather than a result of fibrosis and chronic inflammation.[14–16] Hypoperfusion to the sphincter system of the parotid duct may have relevance in the decreased salivary output of affected glands.[14,15]

TREATMENT
JRP

Even though the acute sialadinitis of JRP is self-limiting, it is important to provide appropriate treatment for palliation and prevention of permanent injury. B-lactam antibiotics (Penicillin VK or Amoxicillin–clavulanate for staphylococcal coverage) can shorten the duration of the symptoms in cases where there is a significant bacterial component. Short-term, low-dose corticosteroid therapy can reduce inflammation and promote faster restoration of glandular function.[2,6–8,15,17] Cannulation of Stenson's duct with lacrimal probes may be useful in breaking adhesions from recurrent infections, as well as clearing precipitated plasma proteins.[2,8] After salivary flow is re-established, sialogogues can be used to prevent further stasis and obstruction. Admistration of a sialogogue in a patient who has an obstructed salivary duct may actually exacerbate an attack. Maintaining hydration will also increase salivary flow and clearance of inflammatory mediators and bacteria. Surgical intervention is rarely necessary in the pediatric population unless there is the formation of an abscess requiring drainage. Because most cases of JRP resolve by adulthood, supportive and prophylactic care is an important aspect in the treatment and management of JRP patients.

Sialendoscopy is a relatively new minimally invasive technique that has shown efficacy in diagnosing and simulatenously treating salivary ductal stenosis, JRP or sialolithiasis. More recent literature reports that interventional sialendoscopy for diagnosed JRP has been efficacious in reducing both acute exacerbations and in preventing future attacks on a long-term basis.[6,8,14–16]

In recent years, evidence supports sialendoscopy with high-pressure saline irrigation as the initial treatment of choice for most cases of JRP or other pediatric and obstructive/restrictive salivary gland diseases. Sialoendoscopes are available with a working diameter of 0.9 mm to 1.3 mm, which can atraumatically enter Stenson's or Wharton's ducts following manual dilation with lacrimal or salivary probes. The endoscope is coupled with irrigation tubing and the duct is continuously irrigated throughout the procedure to maintain patency, which has also proven to be one of the therapeutic advantages of sialendoscopy.[14–16] This procedure can be performed under ambulatory deep sedation/general anesthesia. Recent literature has described the characteristic findings in JRP with endoscopic examination, usually an avascular or hypovascular ductal layer with a distinct white orifice. Sediment from precipitated proteins and bacterial aggregation is observed as a yellowish plaque on Stenson's papilla prior to entering the duct.[14–16] In recent literature, interventional sialendoscopy is proving to be efficacious in treating JRP. The dimensions and placement of the endoscope, alone, can help resolve sialectasis, and high-pressure saline irrigation with or without corticosteroids reduces the incidence of exacerbations and, in many cases, limits recurrence. In areas of the ductal network that are stenotic, balloon dilatation via the endoscopic approach is utilized to maintain the patency of the system and this has been shown to have a long-term therapeutic effect. Sialendoscopy is becoming an the initial treatment of choice for JRP because of its low morbidity and increasingly documented high success rates.[14-16] In 2004, Nahlieli reported a 92% recurrence-free rate of up to 36 months when children with confirmed JRP cases were treated with bilateral sialendoscopy and lavage with intraductal hydrocortisone.[7]

Refractory cases that progress into adulthood may require surgical treatment for improvement or complete resolution. Ductal ligation is a low-morbidity technique that has shown some efficacy in improving symptoms. Tympanic neurectomy of parotid secretomotor fibers can be a useful procedure in denervating the gland and inducing chronic atrophy of the secretory acini but is technique-sensitive. Severing the parasympathetics via the tympanic plexus may not always be enough because some patients have accessory parasympathetic fibers that may run inferior or anterior to the cochlear promontory and may be hidden from the surgical field. Fibers may also course through canals in the temporal bone that are not easily visualized on initial inspection.[18] Vasama reported a 57% symptom-free success rate after neurectomy and 82% of patients in the same study had a marked improvement in symptoms.[19] Parotidectomy is reserved for severely recalcitrant cases of JRP because of the significant morbidity associated with the procedure. There is significant variability in the literature regarding the incidence of permanent facial nerve palsy, but rates range from 10% in trials where only superficial parotidectomy was performed to 100% with total parotidectomy. Resolution of symptoms without recurrence in adult patients with refractory chronic parotitis is remarkable when compared to other less-invasive treatments, but parotidectomy carries a high risk of permanent facial palsy and xerostomia. Becausse this is usually a last-resort treatment for parotitis, there is limited data on the success and morbidity of this procedure on children with JRP.[2,8,15,17,18]

Pneumoparotitis

Pneumoparotitis is swelling and inflammation of the parotid gland secondary to air entrapment or emphysema. Like many other parotid inflammatory conditions, retrograde or ascending air flow into the parotid via Stenson's duct is the initial insult. Pneumoparotid is usually self-limiting because the insufflation of the gland is an acute and usually nonrecurring event. As the excess air slowly exits the parotid gland, swelling and pain decrease the gland returns to its normal state. Often seen following dental procedures from front-exhaust high-speed handpieces that force air through Stenson's duct over the course of several minutes. If enough air is forced into the gland, expansion of the emphysema may traverse the parotidomasseteric fascia and enter into the deep cervical fascia of the neck. Chronic or severe cases of pneumoparotid or pneumoparotitis can result in permanent glandular damage, sialectasis, decreased salivary flow, and fibrosis resulting in frequent/recurrent infections and xerostomia.

At rest, intraoral pressures do not exceed 2–3 mmHg. High speed dental handpieces can raise this to 60 mmHg and activities such as playing reed instruments can create intraoral pressures in the 140–150 mmHg range.[20,21] These high pressure events cause retrograde air flow into the parotid gland via the duct and clinically present as nontender swelling with crepitus, especially if the air has reached the salivary acini, and subcutaneous emphysema if air has escaped the parotid capsule more superficially. There have also been a few reported cases of self-induced pneumoparotid in adolescents either by parafunctional habits or intentionally in children with factious disorders or other psychiatric illness.[20]

Crepitus over the parotid gland is a good indicator of air within the parenchyma, and frothy air filled saliva may be expressed form the duct. There is always the possibility that other fascial spaces of the head and neck will be involved with subcutaneous emphysema and crepitus over the cervical and supraclavicular regions. Noncontrast CT scan is a valuable diagnostic tool and will show diffuse free air within the parotid itself, sometimes making the outline of the gland difficult to see. Stenson's duct will be enlarged and dilated due to the high pressure retrograde airflow, and the extension of the emphysema to other regions of the head and can easily be determined.[22,23]

Bulimia Nervosa Sialadenosis

A very distinct condition afflicting the parotid glands appears in patients with a history of bulimia nervosa, a behavioral eating disorder affecting mostly teenagers and young women. Although bulimia nervosa has only been formally recognized as a disease in the past 30 years, its lifetime prevalence is estimated to be between 4–5%. Bulimia nervosa is characterized by the DSM IV to include recurrent episodes of binge eating paired with inappropriate compensatory behavior to prevent weight gain, the most common being self-induced vomiting. Medical complications of bulimia nervosa include malnutrition, dehydration, hypochloremic alkalosis, gastrointestinal disturbances, hypokalemia, and arrhythmias. At times, the only presenting sign of bulimia nervosa may be a bilateral nonpainful parotid enlargement. The exact pathophysiology of the glandular enlargement is not known, but the most likely explanation is that the recurrent emetic episodes cause an autonomic neuropathy affecting the sympathetic nervous system. The decrease in sympathetic flow to the parotid glands decreases the amount of amylase zymogen granules being secreted and results in an accumulation of enzymes in the acini and gross hypertrophy.[24] Generally, patients have no gross impairment in salivary function but are concerned about the appearance of their facial edema. Parotidomegaly from bulimia nervosa can have a rapid onset and the size of the enlargement be quite impressive.[25]

Most patients with eating disorders are secretive about their habits because of the harsh social stigma associated with it and may not disclose relevant information during a healthcare visit. Although the main clinical implication in bulimic parotidomegaly is of a cosmetic nature, this presentation may be the first chance at recognizing the underlying disease and in helping the patient obtain appropriate consultation and treatment.[26,27]

After recognizing the problem, the most important step is establishing a team-based approach to treat the underlying cause of the disesase. Primary care and psychiatric referral as well as nutritional/metabolic screening are of utmost importance in preventing further complications of bulimia. The unsightly parotid enlargement has been treated successfully in the past by superficial parotidectomy, however, complete resolution of the hypertrophy only occurs if the underlying bulimia and vomiting is controlled.[28,29]

Viral

Mumps is the classic nonsuppurative viral parotitis characterized by localized pain and edema over the parotid glands with associated otalgia and trismus usually occurring in prepubescent childhood. Rarely, the submandibular gland can be affected, but most cases exhibit a unilateral parotitis progressing to bilateral disease. The etiologic agent of mumps is a paramyxovirus, which is spread by airborne droplets from infected saliva and nasal secretions. After entering the respiratory tract, the virus undergoes a 2–3 week incubation period and replicates in the salivary epithelium. Viral prodrome frequently precedes parotitis, which includes typical flu-like symptoms of fever, malaise, arthralgia and myalgia. Orchitis in boys and skin rash may also occur. Currently, the accepted treatment for mumps includes supportive care consisting of hydration, oral hygiene and bed rest. Acidic foods and sialogogues are contraindicated to avoid painful stimulation of the parotids and salivary secretion but has no correlation with decreasing the length of the symptoms. The incidence of mumps in the United States is quite low since the advent and wide administration of the measles, mumps and rubella (MMR) attenuated viral vaccine. Other viruses, such as Coxsackie A and B and Cytomegalovirus have been known to cause viral parotitis but are much less frequent in occurrence. HIV-associated parotitis in children may also be related to an Epstein-Barr virus infection but is clinically mild causing nonpainful enlargement of the parotids. Diagnosis of viral parotitis is usually made by physical exam and history of nonvaccination, but a serum PCR can confirm the diagnosis of mumps.[2,30,31] (see chapters on viral salivary gland infections and HIV-associated salivary gland diseases).

Bacterial

Bacterial or purulent parotitis is a relatively rare disease in children but requires immediate attention and therapy to prevent fascial extension to other head and neck compartments. A 2004 literature review by Spiegel and colleagues reported only 32 cases of acute bacterial parotitis in neonates over the last 30 years. Most of these cases involved premature infants with acute unilateral parotid swelling that were responsive to aminoglycosides and anti-staphylococcal B-lactams for adequate S. aureus and oral flora coverage.[1,32–34] Spiegel reported an approximate 80% cure rate with the preceding treatment regimen. Failure to respond to antibiotics required surgical drainage within 48 hours for satisfactory results.[1]

Mycobacterium tuberculosis infections can rarely involve the parotid glands, which, if untreated, can result in profound glandular dysfunction and destruction. Only 200 cases have been reported in the literature since its first description in 1894.[35] M. tuberculosis, an acid-fast bacillus, is causative for the development of pulmonary tuberculosis and the granulomatous disease of the surrounding lymphatic system.

Because of its waxy mycolic acid coat, ability to survive in macrophages, and other virulence factors, tuberculosis requires a long and aggressive course of antibiotics, even in the absence of clinical presentations. Caseating granulomas within mediastinal and cervical lymph nodes are common, while involvement of parotid lymph nodes and salivary glands rare.[35–37] Several theories have been proposed regarding tuberculosis sialadenitis. After *M. tuberculosis* has colonized a parotid lymph node, it can escape into the parotid parenchyma resulting in a tuberculous sialadentitis. Involvement of the submandibular gland is even less likely to occur.[35,37] Some case reports have shown patients to have primary tuberculous sialadentitis with negative Mantoux skin tests, negative chest radiographs, and negative wound cultures for mycobacterium tuberculosis from associated fistulae that develop on the skin.[36] This may support the theory of an ascending infection via Stenson's duct from colonized tonsillar or oral tissue.[35,37]

Clinically, parotid tuberculosis presents as a slow-growing parotid nodule with intermittent episodes of pain. Fistulae extending to the oral cavity, face, and external ear with purulent drainage have been reported. Cases may mimic salivary gland neoplasms. For this reason, biopsy or fine needle aspiration with cytological examination is imperative in confirming the diagnosis and avoiding unnecessary surgery. MRI and ultrasound may be useful imaging aids in localizing the disease, but they are nondiagnostic and often indistinguishable from a neoplasm. Social history is an important factor in guiding clinicians towards this rare entity. Most cases have been reported on the African or Asian continents and in recent immigrants or travelers from other endemic areas. HIV infection is also a risk factor for any form of tuberculosis and should be taken into consideration.[35–37] Treatment is similar to that of pulmonary tuberculosis and involves multiple antimycobacterial antibiotics for 6 months duration to ensure complete resolution. Without treatment, eventual lymphatic or hematogenous dissemination carries high morbidity and mortality, especially in immunocompromised patients.[35]

DIAGNOSTICS

Sonography is now the most widely used, first line diagnostic tool in detecting pediatric salivary gland pathology. Ultrasound of the parotid gland can effectively reveal hypoechoic and heterogenous areas that correspond to punctuate sialectesis as seen in sialography but with more sensitivity and less time.[2,4,5]

Murrat and colleagues described an imaging algorithm for recurrent parotitis (**Fig. 1**).[38] Ultrasound should also be employed for the initial evaluation for masses, malignancies, cysts, and abscesses in salivary glands because it is a well-tolerated and noninvasive diagnostic procedure. In the emergency department or clinic, ultrasound proves to be a quick, safe, well-tolerated, pain free modality in initial and definitive detection of salivary gland pathology in children.

Sialography is still widely used as a diagnostic tool and is especially sensitive in revealing areas of inflammation, stenosis and obstruction, but its more invasive nature, as compared with ultrasound, has decreased its prevalence as an initial diagnostic method for salivary pathology. The appropriate salivary duct is cannulated with

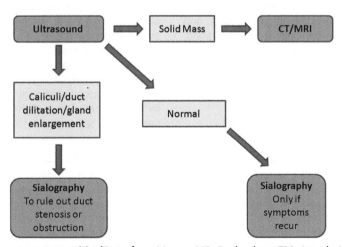

Fig. 1. Algorithm for recurrent parotitis. (*Data from* Murray ME, Buckenham TM, Joseph AE. The role of ultrasound in screening patients referred for sialography: a possible protocol. Clin Otolaryngol Allied Sci 1996;21:21–3.)

a catheter and iohexol, an iodine-based contrast material, is injected into the gland. Galodinium contrast has successfully been used in cases where patients present with iodine allergies. Serial radiographs show retrograde filling of the acini and glandular spaces and are useful in visualizing strictures, filling defects and obstruction. This process requires patient cooperation and can be uncomfortable, so some form of sedation may be required. Typical findings in JRP include punctuate or globular sialectasis of the smaller acinar ducts, which resemble branches of a tree. Some cases display kinks in the main duct, which has been proposed by many to be one of the etiologic factors in JRP. More chronic and long-standing disease may also show sialectasis of larger ducts, but usually no cavitation or filling defects are seen.[4,5,38]

In cases of sialolithiasis, abrupt stoppage or diminished intensity signals proximal to the stone are common, and mass effect from tumors or cysts may present similarly or with displacement and compression of ducts.[17,39] Fibrosis resulting in stricture of the main or larger ducts can be spotted by thin areas of contrast media intensity in the affected system.

CT/MRI

MRI is still considered by many to be the gold standard for detection of salivary gland pathology, especially of the parotid region. Both computerized tomography and MR imaging provide detailed three-dimensional information, and the addition of intravenous contrast media can be helpful in detecting masses, abcesses and arteriovenous malformations. Although MRI and CT have limited clinical practicality in detecting JRP over ultrasound or sialogram, three-dimensional imaging is more sensitive in determining the extent and demarcation of salivary gland inflammation, fibrosis, mass effect or acinar destruction.[2,40,41] Conditions like pneumoparotid can be assessed quickly with a noncontrast CT, and the extent of the trapped air can be evaluated in critical areas without delay.[22,23]

Cytology

Fine needle aspirate is a minimally invasive technique for obtaining a cellular sample of glandular tissue and can provide a quick diagnosis for certain salivary conditions, thereby obviating the need for additional surgical biopsy. Proper technique should be followed to obtain an adequate cellular sample, and this may entail multiple needle passes prior to aspiration of contents for an appropriate smear.[2,35]

Salivary smears from most acutely infected glands of children show similar results: PMN and lymphocytic infiltrate and Gram-positive bacteria, usually *Viridians streptococci* and *S. aureus*. JRP may show some inflammatory cells as well but will likely be lymphocyte predominant.[2,10,42] This is not alone diagnostic for JRP but can help rule out other conditions such as acute bacterial parotitis or salivary tumors. In cases of bulimia nervosa parotidomegaly, FNA and electron microscopy show enlarged acinar cells filled with dark staining granules engorged with amylase zymogen.

Salivary Gland Abscess/Bacterial Sialadentitis

Incision and drainage and antibiotic therapy are indicated in acute salivary gland abscesses. B-lactams with staphycoccal coverage are usually sufficient in most cases as empiric therapy, but incision and drainage of the abscess may be required in patients who do not improve with antibiotics alone within 24–48 hours.[1,32–34,42,43] Because most bacterial infections of the salivary glands originate from oral flora, antimicrobial coverage of staphylococcal and streptococcal species is imperative. Amoxicillin/clavulanate is the drug of choice as empiric therapy as it covers Gram-positive organisms, including staphylococcal species (25–45 mg/kg/day PO divided into two doses for children less than 45 kg). Amoxicillin alone can also be used for uncomplicated infections where staphylococcal species are not implicated. For penicillin allergic patients, clindamycin is appropriate as an alternative (10–25 mg/kg/day PO divided into 3–4 doses, max 1.8 grams per day for children and adolescents). Recurrent bacterial infections and abscesses of the same gland require further diagnostics and appropriate treatment as necessary for possible stricture, obstruction, fibrosis, or sialolithasis. Underlying systemic primary or acquired immunodeficiencies should also be ruled out as for any case of recurrent pyrogenic infections. Retrospective analyses have shown selective IgA deficiency, which is the most common genetic dysgammaglobulinemia, to be implicated in a higher incidence of acute and chronic salivary gland infections and JRP.[44]

Pneumoparotid

Localized pneumoparotid is a self-limiting phenomenon, so identifying and preventing the etiology is critical in limiting recurrence. In cases of recurrent pneumoparotid, the predisposing factor may be a ductal valvular insufficiency where normal increases in intraoral pressures are not tolerated and create spontaneous backflow of air.[22,23] In cases where emphysema extends to fascial planes causing acute respiratory distress or symptomatic pneumomediastinum, decompression may be warranted to remove the trapped air. Slow-resolving pneumoparotid can cause a severe inflammatory response and decreased glandular secretions can result in bacterial superinfection. Cases of infected pneumoparotitis should be treated as a bacterial parotid infection with antibiotics.[1,23]

SUMMARY

The incidence of salivary gland infections in the pediatric population is low but not infrequently seen in pediatric oral and maxillofacial surgery practices and hospital environs. With an ever-increasing armamentarium of diagnostic tools and medical and surgical therapies, these patients can be managed successfully with minimum morbidity and decreased incidence of recurrences.

REFERENCES

1. Stong BC, Sipp JA, Sobol SE. Pediatric parotitis: a 5-year review at a tertiary care pediatric institution. Int J Pediatr Otorhinolaryngol 2006;70(3):541–4.
2. Chitre VV, Premchandra DJ. Recurrent parotitis. Arch Dis Child 1997;77(4):359–63 [Review].
3. Reid E, Douglas F, Crow Y, et al. Autosomal dominant juvenile recurrent parotitis. J Med Genet 1998;35(5):417–9.
4. Sitheeque M, Sivachandran Y, Varathan V, et al. Juvenile recurrent parotitis: clinical, sialographic and ultrasonographic features. Int J Paediatr Dent 2007;17(2):98–104.
5. Shimizu M, Ussmuller J, Donath K, et al. Sonographic analysis of recurrent parotitis in children: a comparative study with sialographic findings. Oral Surg Oral Med Oral Pathol Oral Radiol Endod 1998;86(5):606–15.
6. Nahlieli O, Bar T, Shacham R, et al. Management of chronic recurrent parotitis: current therapy. J Oral Maxillofac Surg 2004;62(9):1150–5 [Review].
7. Nahlieli O, Shacham R, Shlesinger M, et al. Juvenile recurrent parotitis: a new method of diagnosis and treatment. Pediatrics 2004;114(1):9–12.
8. Baurmash HD. Chronic recurrent parotitis: a closer look at its origin, diagnosis, and management. J Oral Maxillofac Surg 2004;62(8):1010–8 [Review].
9. Maynard JD. Recurrent parotid enlargement. Br J Surg 1965;52:784–9.
10. Morales-Bozo I, Urzua-Orellana B, Landaeta M, et al. Molecular alterations of parotid saliva in infantile chronic recurrent parotitis. Pediatr Res 2007;61(2):203–8.
11. Morales-Bozo I, Landaeta M, Urzua-Orellana B, et al. Association between the occurrence of matrix metalloproteinases 2 and 9 in parotid saliva with the degree of parotid gland damage in juvenile recurrent parotitis. Oral Surg Oral Med Oral Pathol Oral Radiol Endod 2008;106(3):377–83.
12. Bernkopf E, Colleselli P, Broia V, et al. Is recurrent parotitis in childhood still an enigma? A pilot experience. Acta Paediatr 2008;97(4):478–82.
13. Kolho KL, Saarinen R, Paju A, et al. New insights into juvenile parotitis. Acta Paediatr 2005;94(11):1566–70.
14. Faure F, Froehlich P, Marchal F. Paediatric sialendoscopy. Curr Opin Otolaryngol Head Neck Surg 2008;16(1):60–3 [Review].
15. Quenin S, Plouin-Gaudon I, et al. Juvenile recurrent parotitis: sialendoscopic approach. Arch Otolaryngol Head Neck Surg 2008;134(7):715–9.
16. Faure F, Querin S, Dulguerov P, et al. Pediatric salivary gland obstructive swelling: sialendoscopic approach. Laryngoscope 2007;117(8):1364–7.
17. Orvidas LJ, Kasperbauer JL, Lewis JE, et al. Pediatric parotid masses. Arch Otolaryngol Head Neck Surg 2000;126(2):177–84.
18. Motamed M, Laugharne D, Bradley PJ. Management of chronic parotitis: a review. J Laryngol Otol 2003;117(7):521–6 [Review].
19. Vasama JP. Tympanic neurectomy and chronic parotitis. Acta Otolaryngol 2000;120(8):995–8.
20. Faure F, Plouin-Gaudon I, Tavernier L, et al. A rare presentation of recurrent parotid swelling: Self-induced parotitis. Int J Pediatr Otorhinolaryngol Extra 2008;4(1):29–31.
21. Ungkanont K, Kolatat T, Tantinikorn W. Neonatal suppurative submandibular sialadenitis: a rare clinical entity. Int J Pediatr Otorhinolaryngol 1998;43(2):141–5.
22. Han S, Isaacson G. Recurrent pneumoparotid: cause and treatment. Otolaryngol Head Neck Surg 2004;131(5):758–61.
23. Luaces R, Ferreras J, Patino B, et al. Pneumoparotid: a case report and review of the literature. Journal of Oral & Maxillofacial Surgery 2008;66(2):362–5 [Review].
24. Mandel L, Abai S. Diagnosing bulimia nervosa with parotid gland swelling. J Am Dent Assoc 2004;135(5):613–6.
25. Vavrina J, Muller W, Gebbers JO. Enlargement of salivary glands in bulimia. J Laryngol Otol 1994;108(6):516–8.
26. Blazer T, Latzer Y, Nagler RM. Salivary and gustatory alterations among bulimia nervosa patients. Eur J Clin Nutr 2008;62(7):916–22.
27. Lo Russo L, Campisi G, Di Fede O, et al. Oral manifestations of eating disorders: a critical review. Oral Dis 2008;14(6):479–84.
28. Burke RC. Bulimia and parotid enlargement–case report and treatment. J Otolaryngol 1986;15(1):49–51.

29. Wilson T, Price T. Revisiting a controversial surgical technique in the treatment of bulimic parotid hypertrophy. Am J Otol 2003;24(2):85–8.

30. Agarwal T, Rahman N, Abel R. Down in the mumps. J Pediatr Surg 2006;41(12):e17–8.

31. Houghton K, Malleson P, Cabral D, et al. Primary Sjogren's syndrome in children and adolescents: are proposed diagnostic criteria applicable? J Rheumatol 2005;32(11):2225–32.

32. Magilner D, Amburgey R. Acute suppurative sialadenitis in a 37-day-old girl. Pediatr Emerg Care 2008;24(4):238–40.

33. Banks WW, Handler SD, Glade GB, et al. Neonatal submandibular sialadenitis. Am J Otol 1980;1(3):261–3.

34. Saarinen RT, Kolho KL, Pitkaranta A. Cases presenting as parotid abscesses in children. Int J Pediatr Otorhinolaryngol 2007;71(6):897–901.

35. Lee IK, Liu JW. Tuberculous parotitis: case report and literature review. Ann Otol Rhinol Laryngol 2005;114:547–51.

36. Alex L, Balakrishnan M, Ittyavirah AK. Tuberculosis of parotid gland - a case report. Indian J Radiol Imaging 2006;16:689–90.

37. Subramanian S, Razak Abdul, Ahmad Faizah. Tuberculosis of parotid gland: a rare differential diagnosis of parotid tumor. The Internet Journal of Head and Neck Surgery 2007;1(2).

38. Murrat ME, Buckenham TM, Joseph AE. The role of ultrasound in screening patients referred for sialography: a possible protocol. Clin Otolaryngol 1996; 21:21–3.

39. Nahlieli O, Eliav E, Hasson O, et al. Pediatric sialolithiasis. Oral Surg Oral Med Oral Pathol Oral Radiol Endod 2000;90(6):709–12.

40. Huisman TA, Holzmann D, Nadal D. MRI of chronic recurrent parotitis in childhood. J Comput Assist Tomogr 2001;25(2):269–73.

41. Sittel C, Jungehulsing M, Fischbach R. High-resolution magneti cresonance imaging of recurrent pneumoparotitis. Ann Otol Rhinol Laryngol 1999;108(8): 816–8.

42. Brook I. Acute bacterial suppurative parotitis: microbiology and management. J Craniofac Surg 2003; 14(1):37–40.

43. Brook I. Suppurative parotitis caused by anaerobic bacteria in newborns. Pediatr Infect Dis J 2002; 21(1):81–2.

44. Fazekas T, Wiesbauer P, Schroth B, et al. Selective IgA deficiency in children with recurrent parotitis of childhood. Pediatr Infect Dis J 2005;24(5):461–2.

Epidemiology of Salivary Gland Infections

Luke Cascarini, BDS, MBBCh, FDSRCS, FRCS[a],*,
Mark McGurk, MD, FDSRCS, FRCS, DLO[b]

KEYWORDS

- Salivary gland infection • Sialadenitis
- Parotitis • Sialolithiasis

Bacterial or viral infections can cause acute or chronic sialadenitis. Sialadenitis of bacterial origin is a relatively uncommon occurrence today and is normally associated with sialoliths. In a study of 877 cases of obstruction, 73.2% were due to salivary calculi and 22.6% were due to salivary stricture formation with no stone present at time of examination.[1]

A hospital study of admissions in the United Kingdom found that the incidence of symptomatic sialadenitis and sialolithiasis was 27.5 and 31.5 per million population respectively.[2] However postmortem studies suggest that the prevalence of salivary calculi might be about 1.2% and they probably form as microcalculi continuously throughout life, being passed spontaneously in most cases without complication.[3]

The most common viral infection of the salivary glands is mumps.

The main factor limiting newer methodologies in, and deeper understanding of, the treatment of salivary disease, appears to be a collective lack of experience. Disorders of the salivary glands are uncommon and, when they occur, experience in managing the process is diluted over a range of disciplines (pediatrics; ear, nose, and throat; general and maxillofacial surgery). The result is that traditional views go unchallenged and are recast unchanged from one textbook to another. This article deviates from this pattern in that sialadenitis is approached on a personal perspective based on 15 years of clinical practice limited mainly to salivary gland diseases.

Ascending acute bacterial parotitis was once a common perimortal event. This is probably because, in advanced disease, the combination of failure to eat and drink leads to dehydration and lack of salivary stimulation, which in combination with immunocompromising comorbidities predispose to infection of the parotid gland by the ascent of oral bacteria. Indeed, President James Garfield died on September 19, 1881, with acute parotitis 2 months after he sustained a gunshot wound followed by several botched procedures that failed to find the projectile.

This scenario is less common today because the advent of antibiotics and improved general hygiene, together with basic modern care, minimize the likelihood of patients becoming very dehydrated.

BACTERIAL INFECTIONS
Acute Bacterial Infections

Acute bacterial sialadenitis is usually caused by bacteria ascending the salivary ducts from the mouth, although bacteremia can occur in the immunocompromised patient. The natural protective barriers to infection are the biologic properties of the saliva, the body's general immune mechanisms, and the physical features of the duct and glandular system. The saliva itself has antibacterial properties and the salivary flow physically washes debris and bacteria out of the duct. It is not widely appreciated that both the submandibular and parotid glands have, in effect, a combination of valves and sphincters to prevent ingress of contaminants.

It follows then that any process that disrupts these natural mechanisms increases the risk of ascending infections. These can be classified as conditions that disrupt the physical flushing effect of saliva through destruction, reduced production

[a] Tonbridge Dental Practice, 155 High Street, Tonbridge, Kent TN9 1BX, UK
[b] Department of Oral & Maxillofacial Surgery, Guy's Hospital, Floor 23, London SE1 9RT, UK
* Corresponding author.
E-mail address: lcascarini@hotmail.com (L. Cascarini).

Oral Maxillofacial Surg Clin N Am 21 (2009) 353–357
doi:10.1016/j.coms.2009.05.004

of saliva, and impact on the protective action of valves and sphincters. Other causes are generalized immunosuppression.

Acute bacterial sialadenitis is more common in the parotid than in either the submandibular or sublingual glands. An explanation for this may be the higher mucoid content of submandibular and sublingual secretions, which protect against bacterial infection. Certainly mucoid saliva contains lysoszyme, which acts by breaking down the 1–4 link between N-acetyl-muramic acid and N-acetyl-glucosamine, which are two of the main bacterial cell wall mucopeptides.[4] Mucoid saliva also contains significant quantities of secretory IgA and, to a lesser extent, IgM and IgD. Mucins also contain sialic acids, which inhibit bacterial attachment to epithelial cells through agglutinating bacteria and glycoproteins.[5] It may also be relevant that the opening of the parotid duct lies opposite the upper second molar teeth, which may be a ready source of bacteria in the unkempt mouth.

Acute bacterial parotitis

By far the most common cause of acute bacterial parotitis is obstruction by calculi or other foreign body. Looking for the cause should be the first line of investigation when confronted by acute bacterial parotitis. Reduced salivary flow in itself is not a strong risk factor and bacterial sialadenitis infection is not a common feature of Sjögren disease. However, reduced salivary flow has increased significance in the presence of other factors, notably immune suppression. Apart from stones, the other factor often associated with acute sialoadenitis is immunosuppression in all its forms. Systemic disorders, such as hepatic and renal disease, and poorly controlled diabetes may precipitate infection as can immunosuppression medication in its more aggressive form (oncology).

Fine needle aspiration of a parotid gland tumor, especially a Warthin tumor, has also been shown to rarely introduce infection[6] and 4% of patients treated by lithography have an acute exacerbation of infection due to the release of bacteria from the shattered calculus.[7]

Causes of reduction in salivary flow may be systemic or local. Systemic factors include dehydration and chemical inhibition of salivary stimulation. Traditionally, local factors include radiation, sialectasis, strictures, tumors, and glandular diseases, such as sarcoidosis and Sjögren disease (**Box 1**).

In practice, the risk of acute infection from these local factors is miniscule. The gland most affected by radiation is the parotid, where salivary flow may

Box 1
Causes of reduced saliva production and flow
Chemical inhibition (see **Box 2**)
Dehydration
Autoimmune disorder
Sjögren disease
Sarcoidosis
Primary biliary cirrhosis
Cystic fibrosis
Renal failure
Infections
Hepatitis C virus
HIV
Extremes of age
Elderly
Neonates
Menopause
Autonomic nervous system dysfunction
Diabetes mellitus
Radiation
Strictures
Stones
Tumors
Iatrogenic damage

be all but eliminated. In most cases, debris or mucoid discharge can be milked from the duct, indicating chronic infection, but acute symptoms are uncommon. Similarly, sialectasis due to chronic obstruction does not lead to acute sialadenitis, but sialectasis arising as a result of repeated infection and destruction of the parenchymal tissues of the gland does indeed represent a significant risk for acute infection. Obstruction by stricture or tumors does not lead to acute symptoms, as saliva on its own is a powerful bacteriostatic agent (ranula and mucocoeles do not frequently become infected). Similarly, acute bacterial sialadenitis is an uncommon event with Sjögren disease and sarcoidosis. Occasionally, patients with advanced Sjögren disease report intermittent painful swelling of parotid glands that seem to respond to antibiotics. A careful inspection of the parotid saliva shows it to be clear. In most of these individuals, the acute swelling and inflammation are due to disregulation of lymphocyte function. A parotid tail biopsy reveals many of these patients to have mucosa-associated lymphatic tissue lymphoma, not recurrent infection. A true bacterial infection of the parotid results in a red, inflamed papilla that stands proud of the buccal mucosa.

The parasympathetic secretomotor innervation of the parotid gland starts in the inferior salivary nucleus and travels in a branch of IX (glossopharyngeal) cranial nerve, which synapses in the otic ganglion acting on nicotinic receptors, and the outflow is via the auriculotemporal nerve, which acts on muscarinic receptors of the gland.

Drugs that attenuate this pathway include anticholinergic drugs, which block atropine and tubocurarine receptors, and drugs that inhibit the release of acetylcholine, such as botulinum toxin (**Box 2**).

Other agents that may reduce saliva production and flow are those that affect the hormonal control of salivary glands. For example, aldosterone increases sodium resorption from the striated ducts and antidiuretic hormone increases water resorption by the striated ducts. Other hormonal influences include thyroxin and testosterone, both of which increase saliva secretion.[4]

Other conditions associated with acute bacterial parotitis include psychiatric disease, probably through a combination of the anticholinergic effects of psychiatric medication as well as anorexia and adipsia associated with depression.

Acute bacterial submandibular sialadenitis

The submandibular duct is prone to obstruction by stones. Most cases of submandibular gland infection are related to this foreign body, which physically has the consistency of coral and is a reservoir for bacteria. In a review of 1200 cases of salivary calculi, 83% were in the submandibular system, 10% in the parotid, and 7% in the sublingual system.[7] Again, other reported causes of infection are tumors, strictures, or iatrogenic damage, such as postsurgery to the floor of mouth or secondary to scarring after trauma to the floor of the mouth. These cause symptoms of obstruction but rarely infection.

Acute minor bacterial sialadenitis

Acute bacterial infection of minor salivary glands is a rare entity. It should be differentiated from other conditions, such as cheilitis glandularis or stomatitis glandularis, which are nonspecific inflammatory conditions. Although secondary infection may play a part in the disease process, it seems not to be the initiating factor. Harold Baurmash in 2003 described three cases of suppurative sialadenitis of the upper lip that were treated by excision of the associated minor glands.[8] Suppurative sialadenitis should not be confused with chronic granulomatous disease.

Box 2
Drugs that cause a reduction in saliva production

Antidepressants

  Tricyclic and selective serotonin reuptake inhibitors

  Lithium

  Bupropion

Alpha-adrenoceptor–blocking drugs

  Antihypertensive drugs and drugs for treating symptomatic benign prostatic hyperplasia

Antihistamines

Antispasmodics

  Baclofen

  Tizanidine

Nicotine replacement therapy

  Bupropion

Centrally acting antihypertensives

  Clonidine

  Methyldopa

  Moxonidine (see alpha blockers above)

Monoamine-oxidase-B inhibitors

Opioids

Appetite suppressants

  Sibutramine

Diuretics

  Any if used excessively

Proton pump inhibitors

  Atropine

Amphetamines

Antipsychotics

Ephedrine

Tetracycline

Botulinum toxin

Steroids

Lead (eg, cases of lead poisoning)

Chronic Bacterial Infections

Chronic bacterial parotitis

True chronic bacterial parotitis is a real entity but is uncommon and overdiagnosed. Due to the chronic nature of bacterial parotitis, there is ample ultrasound evidence of fibrosis and microcyst formation in the gland parenychema. The diagnosis is incomplete without these features being present together with a long history of recurrent, often painful swelling of the parotid gland or glands.

The etiology is multifactorial and may involve a sequence of events that make the gland vulnerable to recurrent infections.[9] The initiating event is usually obscure but Maynard showed that about 30% of children with chronic juvenile parotitis carried the disorder into adulthood.[10] The eventual architectural changes with parenchyma damage and stasis are a prelude to recurrent and persistent infections. This leads to a repetitive cycle of infection, gland damage, and reduction of saliva flow. Accumulation of semisolid material in the ducts causes obstruction of the ductal system and perpetuates the swelling.[11] Saliva is a complex thixatrophic fluid, changing consistency in sympathy with its local environment. Nasal secretions are a good analogy. In the presence of an upper respiratory tract infection, they can be thick and mucoid, but in allergy they can be watery thin. Sialoendoscopy shows that, in the presence of an irritant or stagnation, the saliva clots and forms a gel. This form of saliva predominates in chronic infection.

Chronic recurrent juvenile (parotid) sialadenitis

Chronic recurrent juvenile parotitis is probably not a single entity. One form is caused by a congenital abnormality of the salivary gland ducts. These ducts are large and have a poor seal at the sphincter. Also, the parotid lacks functional value when viewed by sialoendoscope. This results in recurrent attacks of ascending infection.[12] The parotid seems to be the only salivary gland affected. In this group, it is possible to blow air up the parotid duct and sometimes symptoms commence when the child takes up a wind instrument. Children who learn how to induce these symptoms can use them as an excuse to get out of school! Chronic recurrent juvenile parotitis is 10 times more common than adult chronic parotitis[12] and mainly affects children between the ages of 3 and 6, with males being more commonly affected. The symptoms peak in the first year of school, and usually begin to subside around mid-teens. It is unusual for symptoms to persist into the third decade of life. When the disease starts after puberty, females are predominantly affected.[13] When this condition first occurs in childhood, it should be treated aggressively with a protracted course of antibiotics supported by steroids. Anecdotally, this approach reduces the number of cases that transfer to a relapsing course of disease.

Chronic submandibular sialadenitis

Chronic recurrent submandibular sialadenitis Chronic recurrent submandibular sialadenitis is due to incomplete resolution of an acute infection that persists as a chronic relapsing condition, usually because of a failure to treat the underlying cause of the acute infection (eg, removal of the stone). A study of 4600 salivary stones treated at five centers demonstrates that there is usually a delay of 4 to 5 years from first obstructive symptoms (mealtime syndrome) to sialadenitis.[13] Traditionally it is claimed that chronic infection persists even after stone removal because of parenchymal damage leading to stasis and chronic sialolith formation. This view is erroneous. Ten-year follow-up studies now available following lithography demonstrate that glands remain symptom-free as long as the stone is cleared. The recurrent stone rate after removal is approximately 4% of cases.[14] Infection in the submandibular gland almost always involves the sublingual gland. The floor of mouth is firm and a discharge can be milked from the submandibular duct.

Chronic sclerosing submandibular sialadenitis (Kuttner tumor) Chronic sclerosing submandibular sialadenitis is the formation of a painful swollen gland, which is more common in the elderly and mainly involves the submandibular gland although similar processes have been reported in the other major salivary glands. Chronic sclerosing submandibular sialadenitis is associated with sialoliths and nonspecific infectious agents. It is an obscure condition and diagnosis is difficult because of a lack of clear objective criteria.

HIV

HIV-associated salivary gland disease is not an infection of the salivary glands per se but a reaction of the glands to the HIV agent. The resultant enlargement of the glands is termed HIV-associated salivary gland disease. This condition results in reduction of salivary gland function and may lead to secondary ascending infection. The ultrasound appearance is almost diagnostic with the appropriate clinical history. The gland is packed with microcysts, an appearance that is also seen in mucosa-associated lymphatic tissue.

MUMPS

Mumps, a common childhood infection worldwide, is a nonsuppurative infection caused by the mumps virus. It is spread by saliva and urine and typically produces painful swelling of the parotid gland. Complications of mumps include meningitis, encephalitis, thyroiditis, hepatitis, and myocarditis, as well as orchitis and oophoritis, which can affect adults. Other less common complications include deafness and pancreatitis.[15] Apparently in 25% of cases, the salivary swelling may be unilateral, which may serve to obscure the diagnosis unless attention is paid to systemic symptoms.

The condition usually starts with 1 to 2 days of malaise, anorexia and low-grade pyrexia with headache followed by parotid gland enlargement without purulence. The parotid enlargement affects 95% of symptomatic individuals. The swelling progresses over a couple of days and lasts about a week. The orifice of the Stensen duct may be swollen and edematous. In 90% of cases, the contralateral gland is also affected but there may be a time delay between the two sides. In about 10% of cases the submandibular and sublingual glands are affected, which is usually bilateral concomitant with the parotid swelling.[15]

Cerebrospinal fluid pleocytosis occurs in over 50% of cases of mumps, usually without other signs or symptoms of meningitis.[16] Mumps meningitis occurs in 1% to 10% of cases and encephalitis in 0.1%.[16] Epididymo-orchitis affects 15% to 30% of adult males. Five percent of adult females develop oophoritis and mastitis has also been reported. Although mumps meningitis is very benign, mumps encephalitis has approximately 1.5% mortality.[16]

REFERENCES

1. Ngu RK, Brown JE, Whaites EJ, et al. Salivary duct strictures: nature and incidence in benign salivary obstruction. Dentomaxillofac Radiol 2007;36:63–7.
2. Escudier MP, McGurk M. Symptomatic sialadenitis and sialolithiasis in the English population, an estimate of the cost of treatment. Br Dent J 1999;186(9):463–6.
3. Brown JE. Interventional sialography and minimally invasive techniques in benign salivary gland obstruction. Semin Ultrasound CT MR 2006;27(6):465–75.
4. Lavelle CLB. Applied oral physiology. 2nd edition. Chapter 14. Bristol (UK): Wright; 1998. p. 139.
5. Tabak LA, Levine MJ, Mandel ID, et al. Role of salivary mucins in the protection of oral cavity. J Oral Pathol 1982;11:1–17.
6. Bahar G, Dudkiewicz M, Feinmesser R, et al. Acute parotitis as a complication of fine-needle aspiration in Warthin's tumour. A unique finding of a 3-year experience with parotid tumor aspiration. Otolarngol Head Neck Surg 2006;134(4):646–9.
7. Rausch S, Gorlin RJ. Diseases of the salivary glands. In: Gorlin RJ, Goldman HM, editors. Oral pathology. St. Louis (MO): Moseby; 1970. p. 962.
8. Baurmash HD. Suppurative sialadenitis of the upper lip: a report of 3 cases of an infrequent lesion. J Oral Maxillofac Surg 2003;61:1361–5.
9. Motamed M, Laugharne D, Bradley PJ. Management of chronic parotitis: a review. J Laryngol Otol 2003;117(7):521–6.
10. Maynard JD. Recurrent parotid enlargement. Br J Surg 1965;52(10):784–9.
11. Baurmash HD. Chronic recurrent parotitis: a closer look at its origin, diagnosis, and management. J Oral Maxillofac Surg 2004;62:1010–8.
12. Chitre VV, Premchandra DJ. Recurrent parotitis. Arch Dis Child 1997;77(4):359–63.
13. Iro H, Zenk J, Escudier MP, et al. Outcome of minimally invasive management of salivary calculi in 4691 patients. Laryngoscope 2009;9(2):263–8.
14. Zenk J, Bozzato A, Winter M, et al. Extra corporeal shock wave lithotripsy of submandibular stones; evaluation after ten years. Ann Otol Rhinol Laryngol 2004;113(5):378–83.
15. Hviid A, Rubin S, Muhlemann K. Mumps. Lancet 2008;371(9616):932–44.
16. Bang HO, Bang J. Involvement of the central nervous system in mumps. Acta Med Scand 1943;113:487–505.

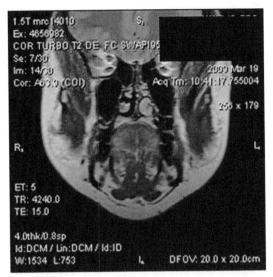

Fig. 1. CT of patient with swelling of her right accessory parotid gland secondary to a relapse of her non-Hodgkin lymphoma.

following: "Within the left submandibular duct, there is a 6.3 mm calcification compatible with a sialolith. Within the left submandibular gland, there is a 2.2 cm × 2.1 cm rim enhancing mass with central low attenuation, compatible with an abscess. The remainder of the left submandibular gland is enlarged and heterogeneous, compatible with sialadenitis."

The final diagnosis was submandibular gland abscess, sialadenitis, and sialolithiasis.

The patient was taken to the operating room for incision and drainage and tolerated the procedure

well, with an uneventful postoperative course. Following resolution of her acute phase, she was scheduled for endoscopic-assisted removal of the sialolith. The sialolith was removed using a sialoendoscopy-assisted sialolithectomy because of the amount of intraductal adhesions. The salivary tissue was observed to be fibrotic and did not appear functional. A salivary stent was placed. One week following, the patient presented back with another submandibular abscess. The decision to perform a sialadenectomy was made. The salivary gland was removed with difficulty secondary to the amount of fibrosis around the gland and the severe inflammation. The postoperative course was noneventful, although she reported increasing xerostomia over the ensuing 6 months. Clinical examination confirmed increasing dryness of the oral mucosa. On a subsequent medical visit, she was diagnosed with Hashimoto thyroiditis (hypothyroidism). Further laboratory evaluation revealed she was positive for SS-A antibodies, and was eventually diagnosed with Sjögren syndrome.

Although Sjögren syndrome is associated with decreased production of saliva and tears, a fibrosis of the parotid glands is generally the major salivary gland most affected. Although the course of treatment would not have been altered in this case, it can be hypothesized that her hypofunction and salivary stasis in her major salivary glands allowed for retrograde migration of oral bacteria, which secondarily contaminated her salivary stone and resulted in fibrosis of her salivary gland tissue. Whether her sialolith formed because of her salivary stasis is unknown.

CASE 3

A 76-year-old woman was consulted for erythematous swelling over the border of the right mandible. Patient was postoperative day 17 from a partial colectomy for the management of an adenocarcinoma located in her large intestine. She developed atelectasis, which progressed into generalized pneumonia. She was currently on "IV antibiotic for the management of pneumonia" at the time of the consult.

Clinical evaluation revealed an enlarged right parotid gland, with overlying erythema. Intraorally, she was edentulous. A small amount of exudate was expressed into her mouth from the Stensen duct. Diagnosis was a right parotid salivary gland infection, "parotitis." CT without contrast was performed confirming an inflamed right parotid gland. No discrete abscess was observed, although the study is limited because contrast could not be administered secondary to her high creatinine.

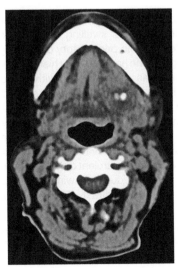

Fig. 2. Seventy-eight-year-old female with a left submandibular swelling and with two sialoliths with fluid collection.

Case Presentations of Salivary Gland Infections

Michael D. Turner, DDS, MD, FACS*, Robert Glickman, DMD

KEYWORDS
- Salivary gland infection • Sialadenitis
- Parotitis • Case reports

Salivary gland infections arise from a wide variety of etiologies: bacteria, localized viruses, systemic viruses, autoimmune diseases, secondary to sialoliths and strictures, and congenital disorders. When dealing with these entities, the diagnosis of the majority of them can be made quickly, although some of the rarer diseases are more difficult to recognize, particularly when they have a more obvious secondary bacterial infection. This article presents six cases and describes their management.

CHIEF COMPLAINT AND HISTORY OF THE PRESENT ILLNESS

Patients generally present with one of two symptoms: (1) swelling of the salivary gland, sometimes painful, sometimes not, or (2) a foul taste in the mouth secondary to purulence. Both of these symptoms may be present concurrently. Clinicians must determine onset, identify precursors to the event, note duration of symptoms, and inquire about past intervention and prior resolutions.

CASE 1

A 54-year-old female presented for evaluation of her enlarged left parotid gland. The patient reported having periodic obstruction of this gland, which resolved over time. She reported significant dryness of her mouth (xerostomia). Past medical history was positive for non-Hodgkin lymphoma, which had been in remission for 3 years. The only pertinent finding on clinical evaluation was poor expression of saliva to palpation of the parotid glands. No exudate was expressed.

Patient was sent for a CT, which revealed: "An irregular enhancing mass in the left buccal space involving the right accessory parotid gland tissue. These findings likely reflect lymphomatous involvement given her history of non-Hodgkin's lymphoma" (**Fig. 1**). Patient was sent to her oncologist for treatment of her relapsing lymphoma.

The past medical history of the patient can be revealing as to the undercurrent diagnosis of the disease process. Autoimmune diseases, diabetes, immunosuppression, or other various diseases must be known at the time of presentation. If patients have recurrent salivary infections, or uncommon features associated with their salivary gland infection, a more extensive workup may need to be initiated.

CASE 2

A 78-year-old female presented emergently with a left submandibular swelling of 1-week duration. The patient had no prior history of swelling or pain in this region. She had a 15-year history of hypertension, which was well controlled with amlodipine 10 mg once daily. There were no other significant findings. On presentation, she was afebrile with a white cell count of 9.1. Her clinical examination was pertinent for a swollen left submandibular swelling, no dysphasia, and no elevation of the floor of the mouth. No saliva or purulent discharge could be expressed from the duct following bimanual palpation. A CT with contrast (**Fig. 2**) revealed the

Department of Oral and Maxillofacial Surgery, New York University College of Dentistry, 345 E. 24th Street, New York, NY 10010, USA
* Corresponding author.
E-mail address: docturner@nyu.edu (M.D. Turner).

Oral Maxillofacial Surg Clin N Am 21 (2009) 359–362
doi:10.1016/j.coms.2009.05.005

Infectious disease consult advised to add vancomycin. The patient expired 5 days later secondary to respiratory failure.

Postsurgical parotitis is an ominous finding, particularly in the elderly. Its incidence is reported to be 0.02% to 0.04% and usually presents 1 to 15 weeks following surgery, although it has a peak incidence of between postoperative days 5 and 7, and is associated with a mortality rate of approximately 25%. This mortality rate serves as an indicator of poor prognosis following surgery, but is rarely the primary cause of death. Postsurgical patients develop parotid gland infections because of their dehydration, which allows for a retrograde microbial migration. Patients with chronic illness also can have poor nutrition, as well as systemic compromise to their all-around general health.

Recent past surgical history is very important when dealing with salivary gland infections. In head and neck oncology patients, radiation to the tumor or postresection site causes fibrosis of the parotid glands within 2 to 6 months, depending on the dosage and the field of radiation. There is not a high incidence of salivary gland infections in these patients probably because of the concurrent fibrosis of the gland and the duct, which prevents retrograde microbial contamination. When a salivary gland infection does occur in this region, treatment is difficult, either medically or surgically. Because the gland is fibrosed and hypovascular, penetration of the antibiotic to the infected region is difficult. Hyperbaric oxygen may be considered for its angiogenic properties, although this is hypothetical because this scenario is rare. Such a salivary gland infection should not be confused with radiation-induced parotitis, which is an inflammation of the gland and resolves following the completion of radiation treatment. Antibiotic treatment is not indicated for this condition.

CASE 4

A 45-year-old female presented for evaluation of an extremely painful left parotid gland. This was a first-time occurrence for her. Medical history revealed no abnormalities requiring further investigation. Clinical evaluation was positive for an enlarged left parotid gland, which was painful to palpation. No exudate was expressed. Patient was sent for CT, which showed generalized parotitis.

Patient started to have resolution of swollen left parotid when her right parotid began to swell (**Fig. 3**). It appeared to be an adult case of mumps, although patient had received appropriate vaccinations as a child. The patient had been in Uganda

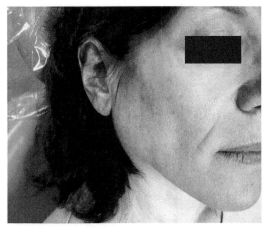

Fig. 3. Adult patient presenting with sialadenitis secondary to mumps.

1 month prior. A sample of a small amount of expressed saliva was sent to laboratory for ELISA, which confirmed the diagnosis of mumps.

As previously discussed, mumps presents 90% of the time in the parotid gland and 70% bilaterally. The parotid swelling is asymmetric at onset, reaching maximum proportion in 2 to 3 days. The infection is spread through respiratory droplets, resulting in a viremia 12 to 25 days later, which lasts from 3 to 5 days. It can spread to meninges, other salivary glands, the pancreas, testes, and ovaries. Recent outbreaks have led to the hypothesis that there may be a waning vaccine-induced immune response, and that lifelong immunity might not be assured as previously thought. Evidence shows that vaccinated individuals and possibly also naturally infected individuals might become more susceptible with time following the last exposure to the mumps virus.

CASE 5

A 14-year-old male presented with a swollen right parotid gland (**Fig. 4**). The patient had a history of both parotid glands "swelling up" since he was 8 years old. He had been evaluated by a variety of physicians, who generally gave him antibiotics. The swelling generally resolved over 1 or 2 days. He had no other significant medical history. His two brothers and one sister did not have these symptoms.

Juvenile recurrent parotitis is the second most frequent pediatric salivary gland cell disease next to mumps. Generally, patients are prepubert and the disease affects only the parotid glands and is generally bilateral. The exact etiology of the disease has been hypothesized to be congenital, although further study needs to determine if the

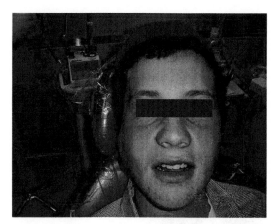

Fig. 4. Fourteen-year-old male with juvenile recurrent parotitis.

occurrence is triggered by an unknown viral infections (personnel correspondence, James Melville). The treatment in the past has ranged from frequent use of antibiotics to surgical intervention, such as superficial parotidectomy, ligation of the parotid duct, and tympanic plexus neurectomy. Generally, until the onset of sialoendoscopy, these treatments had limited effectiveness while putting the patient at risk for facial nerve injury, parotid abscess, and other long-term consequences of surgery. Sialoendoscopic management is generally successful, but there are cases that fail this intervention. Juvenile recurrent parotitis generally resolves in patients following puberty, although it can persist into adulthood. Questions persist about whether this disease entity in the past was misdiagnosed as mumps, and whether the adult form of chronic parotitis is related to, and possibly triggered by, various forms of hyposalivation (eg, pharmacy-induced hyposalivation).

CASE 6

A 62-year-old male presented with recurrent enlargement of his right parotid gland. The patient reported a 20-year history of drainage of purulent exudate from the duct. The gland remains constantly swollen. He reported that when the gland became painful, he would take various antibiotics, which resolved the discomfort but did not change the size of the gland or the discharge from the duct.

He had no significant past medical history. CT was consistent with chronic parotitis. Patient was taken to the operating room for exploration and drainage of his salivary gland. Significant fibrosis and adhesions were seen. Microdissection of the duct and lysis of adhesions were performed. Following postoperative healing, patient symptoms and signs were normal for 4 months, during

which time he had no notable purulent drainage, and the parotid gland decreased to a normal size. At approximately 4 months postoperatively, the patient had another episode of swelling and pus. The patient was taken back to the operating room, where he had more lysis of adhesions and irrigation of the gland duct system. The patient remains asymptomatic 4 years following initial surgery, with normal serous saliva from the gland.

Chronic salivary gland infections are by no means easy to manage. Significant damage to the gland from bacteria causes severe fibrosis, which in cyclical fashion, worsens the infection, which then can lead to more fibrosis. These infections persist for years. However, owing to their constant drainage from the ducts, pus does not collect and form a discrete abscess. If the ductule system becomes obstructed, pus accumulates. Generally, these cases are initially treated with long, multiple courses of antibiotics, with asymptomatic periods and relapse. With increasing frequency of obstructive occurrences, sialadenectomy of the submandibular gland or a superficial parotidectomy is often performed. Removal of the submandibular gland is curative. The removal of the superficial lobe of the parotid gland is generally curative, although symptoms can persist because of the retention of the deep lobe of the parotid. Depending upon the severity and duration of the chronic infection, dissection of the superficial lobe from the facial nerve can be difficult because of the severe inflammation and scarring of the region.

Sialadenectomy should be considered the treatment of last resort when managing chronically infected salivary glands. The initial step should be evaluation of the etiology of the problem, either localized obstruction or systemic disease. The type of localized obstruction should also be determined. If obstruction is secondary to a sialolith, the stone should be either fragmented, removed, or both as indicated. If the obstruction is secondary to scarring either from an acute salivary gland infection (bacterial, viral, or other), reestablishment of an intraoral drainage path can be effective and may obviate further surgery. Once the primary outflow of the ductule system is patent, determination as to the function of the gland can then be determined. Anecdotally, in cases of salivary infections in conjunction with sialolith, once the stone is removed, the patients generally become asymptomatic, even in cases where the gland is completely fibrosed and nonfunctional. If infection persists after a stone is removed and/or the ductule system is created, the indication for the removal of the gland is more reasonable.

Index

Note: Page numbers of article titles are in **boldface** type.

Oral Maxillofacial Surg Clin N Am 21 (2009) 363–367
doi:10.1016/S1042-3699(09)00065-X

oralmaxsurgery.theclinics.com

Moving?

Make sure your subscription moves with you!

To notify us of your new address, find your **Clinics Account Number** (located on your mailing label above your name), and contact customer service at:

E-mail: elspcs@elsevier.com

800-654-2452 (subscribers in the U.S. & Canada)
314-453-7041 (subscribers outside of the U.S. & Canada)

Fax number: 314-523-5170

Elsevier Periodicals Customer Service
11830 Westline Industrial Drive
St. Louis, MO 63146

*To ensure uninterrupted delivery of your subscription, please notify us at least 4 weeks in advance of move.

Our issues help you manage *yours.*

Every year brings you new clinical challenges.

Every **Clinics** issue brings you **today's best thinking** on the challenges you face.

Whether you purchase these issues individually, or order an annual subscription (which includes searchable access to past issues online), the **Clinics** offer you an efficient way to update your know how...one issue at a time.

DISCOVER THE CLINICS IN YOUR SPECIALTY!

Dental Clinics of North America.
Publishes quarterly. ISSN 0011-8532.

Oral and Maxillofacial Surgery Clinics of North America.
Publishes quarterly. ISSN 1042-3699.

Atlas of the Oral and Maxillofacial Surgery Clinics of North America.
Publishes biannually. ISSN 1061-3315.

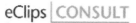

Where the Best Articles become the Best Medicine

Visit **www.eClips.Consult.com** to see what 180 leading physicians have to say about the best articles from over 350 leading medical journals.

M022487

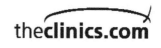

Printed and bound by CPI Group (UK) Ltd, Croydon, CR0 4YY

03/10/2024

01040352-0012